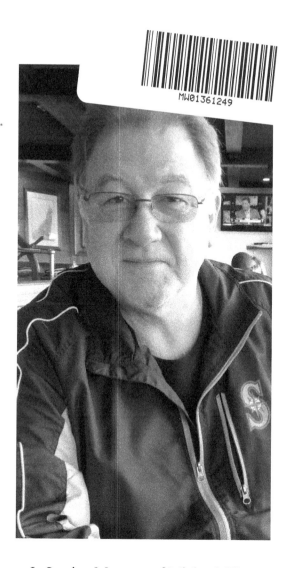

In Loving Memory of Michael Cline
Devoted Father & Loving Husband
Respiratory Therapist, College Instructor, Author
January 25, 1956 – March 10, 2018

FOREWORD

On March 10th, 2018, only a few weeks before the official conclusion to the publishing of this book, Michael Cline, my beloved father, and the author of this memoir, unexpectedly passed away at his home in Tacoma, Washington. His untimely death came as a tremendous shock to my family and I, not to mention his numerous colleagues in the healthcare world, and to the hundreds of patients and students that currently were, or had previously been, under his care and instruction throughout his forty plus years of working in respiratory therapy. The intellectual and professional void left behind from his sudden departure can never again be filled, and his incredible legacy as a respiratory therapist and a teacher will never be forgotten.

To call my father a "master of his craft" would be an understatement. Over the course of his life he devoted hundreds of hours, both on the job and off, towards learning all about the delicate intricacies and medical functions of the human lungs, towards understanding and utilizing the many different forms of respiratory equipment used in the field of respiratory homecare, as well as towards refining the techniques and interpersonal approaches towards proper patient care. Anyone who knew him personally would say that he was not only an unmatched wunderkind of the respiratory world, but a gentle soul and a humble gentleman who was deeply passionate about improving the lives of his many patients, and who took great pride in helping people "learn to breathe all over again".

Since his passing, I have worked with the staff at Olympia Publishers to finalize the publishing of this book. Prior to his death, my father had finished writing every short story that he wished to have included in his memoir, and all that remained was proofreading, cover approval, and the eventual printing. Other than the inclusion of this foreword, an afterword, and some letters of acknowledgment from colleagues who knew Michael Cline and who offered to voice their support for the publishing and promotion of this book, I have left my father's original work entirely untouched, to and including his original "About the Author" page.

Whether you are reading this book for pleasure, to learn more about my father's legacy, to improve upon your own skills and overall understanding of respiratory care, or perhaps even as part of some professional RT development course or medical college curriculum, I deeply hope that you will enjoy reading this book and that some of my father's many years worth of respiratory therapy wisdom will be "breathed" into you in the process.

In loving memory of my father, the greatest man I ever knew.

Christopher M. Cline

Acknowledgment for a Life of Service

With honor, I express a celebration of Mike Cline's professional respiratory skills and friendship. His always-pressing positive attitude, genuine dedication and compassion to his patients and students and, in my case, his professional peer for over twenty-five years of collaboration in the ever changing world of hospital to home respiratory care.

Mike Cline shared his rich and classic respiratory knowledge with unconventional wisdom and an amazing sense of humor. His genuine willingness and great pride in his craft fill the pages of this book with thoughtful and insightful story telling. Readers of this volume from all fields of healthcare may see parities in their own daily experiences, including not to take oneself too seriously. This book will be enjoyed by both young and old respiratory students as well those whom Mike termed as the lifelong learners through engaging the experiences of others.

Mike's professional career shrouded a sense of history in the beginning of what was then known as the original Inhalation Therapy techniques. His strong understanding and expert knowledge of the initial tools available to clinicians of that day—much less sophisticated mechanical negative pressure ventilation, IPPB and the omnipresent hand bagging techniques was his foundation. Many improvements in respiratory equipment technology have changed the field and led to amazing patient outcomes pioneered by many individuals and the American Association of Respiratory Care which Mike was not only a member, but an ardent supporter and advocate to his trade. As exciting as these new methods are, today's better clinical understanding of the pathophysiology of mechanical ventilation has led to more humanistic approaches to respiratory patient care and intervention protocols.

Mike was sensitive to the toll facing both patients and clinicians today and well adept to the simple but ever important sounds of breathing, providing the needed patient comfort and confidence. He was a highly regarded resource for numerous physicians garnering exceptional respect and trust. As a peer for his fellow R.T.'s Mike was a leader, a confidant, and always in the moment, yet ready to lighten any load through hard work and a dose of humor with great integrity. These qualities can hardly be replaced and my sincerest hope is that by reading this book we take a piece away from Mike Cline's life and best practices to appreciate not only the respiratory profession, but a life well lived to the benefit of so many. Mike was my friend and my teacher.

Mark Kuipers
Vice President
Performance Home Medical

Acknowledgment for a Legacy of Teaching

I met Mike Cline sixteen years ago when I began working with Tacoma Community College's Respiratory Care program. At that time, Mike's primary responsibility with the college was teaching respiratory equipment and a survey of science class, which included information on chemistry, microbiology, and physics as it related to the respiratory therapy field. Mike was a talented instructor who had a tremendous gift for being able to transform very difficult, complex subject matter into information that was easier for students to understand. His detailed drawings on the white board enlightened key concepts, and his unique ability to tell "war" stories from his many years of experience as a respiratory therapist, were just a few of the techniques Mike employed to bring the message across. Students often looked forward to Mike's Friday morning class where they were greeted by Mike's jovial easygoing demeanor and the dozens of doughnuts Mike would often bring.

Mike was much more than a professor of Respiratory Therapy. Mike was also a mentor to the many people who knew him. He demonstrated what it took to be a professional in the field he loved and enjoyed for over forty years. He was a strong advocate for the respiratory profession but most importantly to the patients he served.

Mike's passing will certainly leave a big void at Tacoma Community College and the surrounding respiratory community. Mike was one of a kind. He will be missed, but definitely not forgotten. This book will ensure Mike's legacy as a respiratory instructor and story teller will live on for years to come. This book unfolds amazing stories of Michael Cline's forty years as a respiratory care practitioner. It will impart a small glimpse into what occurred every Friday morning, for twenty plus years in the allied health building at Tacoma Community College when Mike took to the lectern teaching the future respiratory therapists of Washington State. We hope you enjoy Mike's stories and his knowledge as much as we did.

Thank you Mike for sharing your wisdom and knowledge to the many students who have been a part of the TCC Respiratory Program. Your dedication to the profession and the program have contributed to the many exceptional Respiratory Care Practitioners who have graduated from Tacoma Community College. We're going to miss you.

Greg Carter,
M.Ed. RRT Program Director,
Tacoma Community College Respiratory Program

Acknowledgment for a History of Compassionate Patient Care

Michael Cline is a truly great storyteller. In this book, he tells the stories of patients he has served over his forty-year respiratory therapy career, along with a few other great tales. If you're looking for intimate, informative, inspirational, entertaining, poignant, surprising and funny stories, *In the Ocean of Air* is the book for you. Any person affected by a lung disease, whether they are a patient, caregiver, physician, nurse, respiratory therapist, or social worker, will truly enjoy this book and learn from it. But Michael spins such terrific tales, that anyone looking for an entertaining read will enjoy his stories.

Michael and I met when I was being fitted for a CPAP, something I wasn't sure was for me. He convinced me to give it a try and in the process we bonded instantly. I had gained a new friend and as a bonus, the CPAP worked.

He was very interested in my story. I was diagnosed with Idiopathic Pulmonary Fibrosis in 2004 and received a double lung transplant in 2006. Here it is 2018 and I'm still alive and kicking. Since my transplant I've been able to lead three support groups for IPF and Lung transplant patients, and have become very involved as the Chairman of the Pulmonary Fibrosis Foundation for several years. I've had a window into the lives of several hundred patients struggling with lung disease and with the challenges of becoming listed for, waiting for, surviving and thriving after a lung transplant. Michael does a particularly good job of describing the agonizing wait and the transformation of patients after receiving new lungs.

Michael asked me to share my experience with Idiopathic Pulmonary Fibrosis and the lung transplant that has given me twelve additional high quality years with the Pulmonary Rehabilitation students at Tacoma Community College. It was instantly apparent that these students admired and appreciated Michael Cline. This book is a gift to them and anyone who wants to be informed and inspired by his stories.

His descriptions of the various lung diseases he saw as a respiratory therapist are easily understood by anyone. He creates a visual image of what is happening inside the human body, turning the technical descriptions of physicians into mental images that patients can understand. This book is full of great stories, mostly about real people who have faced fatal disease with courage, dignity, persistence, strength, resilience, and above all, humor and a positive attitude.

Michael does a great job of building each character in his stories. It makes them easy to relate to as they go through their own life adventures. Some adventures are medical and some are just plain interesting and fun. They are all real people and you'll love his characters as much as he does. They are his heroes.

Enjoy this book. It is a labor of true love!

Michael Henderson
Former Chairman
Pulmonary Fibrosis Foundation

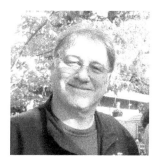

Michael W. Cline
Registered Respiratory Therapist
BS in Health Sciences in Professional Development and Advanced Patient Care
Homecare Respiratory Therapist, Performance Home Medical, Kent, WA.
Adjunct Faculty Member Respiratory Therapy Program Tacoma Community College

About the Author

Mike has been a respiratory therapist since 1976, and has instructed at Tacoma Community College for over twenty years. Throughout, he has been a licensed pilot, a certified scuba diver, a licensed real estate agent, and a stay-at-home dad—at which time, he published a manual on wood strip boat building. But despite the many spin-offs and elusive dreams and schemes, respiratory therapy held serve as his occupation. Now, if not writing, teaching, or working in respiratory therapy, Mike is man of basic needs and simple pleasures. He enjoys breathing oxygen and exhaling carbon dioxide, and yearns to do so perpetually. He lives in Tacoma with his wife Tara, and has two children, Chris and Kaela.

In the Ocean of Air

Stories and Adventures from Forty Years of Respiratory Care

Michael W Cline

In the Ocean of Air

Stories and Adventures from Forty Years of Respiratory Care

Olympia Publishers
London

www.olympiapublishers.com
OLYMPIA PAPERBACK EDITION

Copyright © Michael W Cline 2018

The right of Michael W Cline to be identified as author of
this work has been asserted in accordance with sections 77 and 78 of the
Copyright, Designs and Patents Act 1988.

All Rights Reserved

No reproduction, copy or transmission of this publication
may be made without written permission.
No paragraph of this publication may be reproduced,
copied or transmitted save with the written permission of the publisher,
or in accordance with the provisions
of the Copyright Act 1956 (as amended).

Any person who commits any unauthorised act in relation to
this publication may be liable to criminal
prosecution and civil claims for damage.

A CIP catalogue record for this title is
available from the British Library.

ISBN: 978-1-78830-046-9

This book is about real people and real events that are imbedded in my personal health care experiences. No family names are mentioned and no sensitive HIPAA information is revealed in any of the general discussions of the medical scenarios. The few first names that appear in the stories are those of long-term RT compatriots who won't have a problem being mentioned. And the only full name divulged in one of the stories is that of Joe Morton, and to return the facetious, now forty-four-year-old sentiment—no one cares what that clown thinks.

First Published in 2018

Olympia Publishers
60 Cannon Street
London
EC4N 6NP

Dedication

I would like to dedicate this book to all the Respiratory Therapists who ever were, including my own father. He retired from the army after twenty-four years of service in 1971. He then went to St. Joseph's Hospital / Tacoma Community College (TCC), to become an "Inhalation Technician." (The original IT acronym!) After I graduated from high school in 1974, he encouraged me to get a skill first, by going to respiratory school. But I resisted and went off to study Biology at Rocky Mountain College in Montana. He was a Certified Respiratory Therapy Technician (CRTT) at St Joe's, and my mother (Sally Cline) was a Registered Nurse at Tacoma General Hospital, and my life was plumb full of hospital, dinner-table talk at the time. A year later, my father asserted, "you've got one year of college now, but you still don't have a skill. You need to get a skill to fall back on for the future." Still I resisted, and went a second year of college locally at TCC itself, where I concentrated on classes bent toward a Biology degree, and was able to play one last year of college baseball. I thought maybe I would be a Biology teacher (maybe go back and teach at Bellarmine High School, as other alums have done), or maybe try to get into medical school at some point. Either way, science of some sort was my proclivity. After my second year was completed, my father tersely reminded me, "now you've got two years of college and you still don't have a skill. You need to get a skill! Plus, you can pick up a lot of science credits along the way! Plus, you can get a job anywhere, and work at a hospital while you are completing your education!" He drove a hard bargain at that point. So, I looked at the curriculum and decided that, indeed, becoming a respiratory therapist would add a skill and enhance my science credits toward completing a Bachelor's degree. So, I started respiratory therapy school in June 1976. And, looking back, it was no doubt the best advice that I was ever relentlessly coerced to take! Perhaps, in a later book, the gangly topic of working in the same field and in the same place as a parent, with its humorous foibles and pitfalls can be elucidated.

But for now, both mom and dad are long at rest, so I will posthumously thank Dad for his persistent fatherly advice, and, again, cast a wide dedication and kudos to all the RTs out there, who know what it is like to have a real job! Especially those who ever spent a shift working with the ineffable Bill Cline.

Contents

Introduction 21

Don't Sit Under the Bacon Tree with Anyone Else but Me 25

The Tragedy of Tripping Hazards and Fatal Falls in the Home 41

Trading Places. In the Morgue 47

Rookie Mistakes in Respiratory Care 56

Medical Incompetence and Opportunities for Improvement ...or Skipping Town? 66

You Only Live Once. The Uproarious Caper of the Boot Camp Banjo 78

Hospital Workplace Violence and the Many Shades of Code Orange 88

A Demonic Encounter: A Patient Deeply Possessed of Mind and Numerous Bullet Fragments 106

Love You to Death. Until We Do Part 117

The Nexus of Wolff-Parkinson-White Syndrome and a
Discounted Refrigerator Repair Job 125

Obstructive Sleep Apnea, American Cyanide, and the
Downfall of Nazi Germany 134

Microsoft Windows (Obstructive) Sleep (Apnea) Mode
and Other Off-Campus CPAP Adventures 148

Happy Endings. The Complex Sleep Apnea Gremlin,
the Distraught Lawyer, the Angry Judge and the
Triumphant Gremlin Busters 160

A Short Primer on Children, Sleep Apnea, CPAP and the
Preternatural Flight of REM Boy! 175

Campomelic Dysplasia and a Beautiful but
Abbreviated Childhood 183

The Glory to Shine a Second Time. Lung Transplantation,
Organ Donation and The Gift of Life 191

Diane's story. Go Dawgs! And the flight of the
hummingbird. 196

Sheila's story. "As long as you have breath, there is hope."
And the Clash of the Sibling Beauties 204

He's number one! The Uproariously Hypoxic Life
and Times of "Ex-Vivo" Ed 215

Introduction
The Ocean of Air, the Ocean of Life

As earthly humans, we all live at the bottom of an ocean of air. This fluid ocean has great waves, whirlpools and currents running through it. Birds, bats and insects easily swim and dart around in it, while pollens, spores and dandelion seeds slowly drift and float like plankton in it. Speeding pebbles from outer space routinely penetrate the uppermost surface of it. Some of the larger meteors may reach the ground, but most plunge and burn away into the lower thick of it. And, also similarly to the watery ocean, our ocean of air has lunar and solar tides that cyclically alter the depth, temperature and mixture of it.

In composition, our gaseous ocean is twenty-one per cent oxygen (O_2), seventy-eight per cent nitrogen (N_2) with one per cent trace gases of Argon, Neon, CO_2, Helium, Hydrogen, and several others. Most importantly, the robust and chemically reactive oxygen content makes the ocean of air very corrosive, acid-forming, and highly supportive of combustion. Consequently, the modern, universal chemical term for burning is *"oxidation."* However, the very term *oxy-gen* originated from an ancient, wine-brewer's word meaning *"acid-maker."* It was fully known to vintners that a mysterious substance in the air would turn one's vintage into *vinegar* if the fermentation vat wasn't airtight. (The word *vinegar* itself is Old French for *sour wine*).

Of greatest consequence to our human existence, this omnipresent oxygen content also makes the ocean of air highly supportive of life, all across every landmass and dissolved into the depths of all bodies of water. Deep down in cyclopean blackness, sea creatures, nestled within the wreckage of the Titanic, sift atmospheric oxygen through their gills. The ocean of life-sustaining air reaches deep.

Of all the attributes and vulnerabilities that we share as human beings, by far the most vital is the immediate need for oxygen. One can live for days without water, weeks without food, but not six minutes without oxygen. Oxygen is the singular vital nutrient that has no storage capacity whatsoever. It is absorbed and utilized by tissue cells as fast as the hemoglobin can deliver it. There is no reserve pool of oxygen, to speak of, for the body to fall back on. Ultimately, we cannot leave our oxygen-rich ocean for an instant, and astronauts who venture into the void of space beyond, must take a large, compressed bubble of the ocean with them. And when a sick patient on earth requires more oxygen than is currently available to them in the atmosphere, the Respiratory Therapist (RT) intervenes with various devices that will facilitate an *alternate inspiratory atmosphere* commensurate to that patient's clinical needs. This is no small responsibility; the astute RT will be counted upon to make keen assessments of a patient's clinical status, to recommend the appropriate therapy and to set up and operate the proper equipment.

In the forty years during which I have been associated with the Respiratory Therapy profession, I have worked for hospitals, home care companies, and health care agencies; and I still currently teach part time in the Respiratory Therapy Program at Tacoma Community College. I have seen a lot of changes in the health care workplace, in healthcare practices, and in the remarkable evolution of life-saving equipment. But the ultimate experience is the opportunity to work closely and personally with people who need your help. And I have found that working with people up close lends to a personal enrichment that needs to be shared.

This collection of stories is an eclectic mixture of my personal experiences in the respiratory healthcare field. They are somewhat personally chronological, but not meant to be a full memoir—they are mostly bent on providing a human touch, be it educational, emotional, or just plain fascinating. Some stories are tragic, some are tremendously uplifting, and at least few are hilarious in their own right. Ultimately it is all about people. People whom you meet, and have the opportunity to help. People are amazing, people are quirky and people are prone to tragedy and triumph in ways never anticipated. As an example, in the lead story, the most remarkable human beings you will ever meet are not on television. They are behind windows and doors of anonymous houses along the road where they are enduring enormous sacrifice in the long-term care of an afflicted family member and maintaining an inspiring and upbeat attitude about it all. Bad things happen to good people, and it is amazing to see how good people don't let the bad things alter who they are. And, on top of that, life always finds a way to be amazing further still. I hope you enjoy these stories, and maybe gain some pearls of wisdom, laughter and appreciation for the life we share together in our great Ocean of Air.

Don't Sit Under the Bacon Tree With Anyone Else but Me

The Magnificent Trailblazer and the Distraught Honeymooners

This heartbreaking and yet beautifully uplifting and humorous story is right off the great carousel of life. This is the unlikely story of two respiratory homecare patients of mine who were not the least bit related to each other, but coincidentally had a very heart-warming mutual connection between them. The two families lived about three miles apart, just off the same East-West thoroughfare in the Kirkland, WA area. It was pure serendipity that I stumbled on to the connection between the families, and it yet again demonstrates that you just never know what can develop when you are deeply involved with people's private lives and their personal health care. And it is yet another sterling example of the ineluctable human amenities to be experienced when working in the field of home health care.

The first patient in this scenario was a stellar and accomplished gentleman who was stricken with Amyotrophic Lateral Sclerosis (Lou Gehrig's disease), and was now bedridden and ventilator-dependent. He had traveled the world as an aerospace executive and was a lifelong outdoor enthusiast, having climbed most of the world's major peaks, except for Everest. He was highly philanthropic, and was active in the community on many levels. The dismal lament about the bad things that happen to good people could not be more applicable. This exceptional man was the last person whom one would ever want to see beset with a degenerative neuromuscular condition that slowly paralyses the body completely, while leaving the mind at full acuity. When I took over his respiratory home care, he was nearing end-stage, fully bed-ridden with a tracheostomy, but was currently able to communicate with his still-active right hand. His wife had made a small alphabet card, and had clipped it to the bed rail, where he could dutifully poke his index finger at the letters and spell out the words of conversation. Many months later, when his hand muscles atrophied, the wife came up with a new communication strategy that she learned from an Occupational Therapist. She used a large poster board with a hole cut out of the middle for her face to fit through. Stationed concentrically around the hole were both letters of the alphabet and further out (compass fashion) were whole words like bedpan on the right, suction on the left, oral care on top and so forth. By facing him from the foot of the bed, with her own face in the poster, she could watch the articulation of his eyes and quickly ascertain which words or letters his eyes were looking at, and then act accordingly. It was a truly remarkable and effective silent communication tactic, and occupational therapists are worth their weight in gold when it comes to conceptualizing workable solutions like this for highly-challenged patients at critical disease stages. (When it comes to ingenious health care tactics and self-help devices that cause you to inquire, "Who even thinks of this kind of stuff?" very often the answer is an Occupational Therapist; it is a meticulous and multifaceted vocation that no one can summarize.)

I had worked with this magnificent man for not quite two years, and in the several finger-poke conversations I had shared with him, the sentinel discussions involved the life activity that he cherished most. Going way back to the early nineteen-fifties, as a young man he had been one of the original members of the (still active) Trail Blazers Club. The original group had started teaching people hiking safety, survival skills, and helping to blaze trails all throughout the Cascades for hiking and camping enthusiasts. And one of his most beloved pioneering projects (still carried on by members today) was the stocking of brook trout in the high, remote alpine lakes region. Back in the fifties, they carried heavy metal water tanks filled with trout fry on their backs and hoofed them up some mighty precarious trails, often inching along sheer drop-offs, and scooting around cliff ledges and the like. And in that daring regard, there was one particularly difficult mountainous area that held a special place in his heart. It was the Jewel Lakes region in the central Cascades. The Jewels are a string of several small lakes that are suspended in a high alpine valley (aptly named the Necklace Valley.) Surrounded by jagged hillsides and cliff walls, this area was not easy to get to, and was by no means a trek for beginners. In the early 1950s, after stocking the Jewels with trout, beside one of the lakes they constructed a small, quaint wood cabin for the public to use. They affixed to the cabin a brass plaque, as a testimonial to the Trail Blazers Founder and Credo. And the essential, Good Samaritan sentiment was that any hikers with the gumption to get past the spooky parts of this already steep, tiresome, nine-mile ascent would have a nice little shelter to stay in for their efforts. How cool is that? Those were the days.

Everything about this wonderful man was wholesome and emulative and inspiring. It was an honor to have known him, and God knows that this often-troubled world could use so many more like him. And that equally applies to his selfless and ever-attentive wife, who was there night and day, exhausting every last communication technique available to maintain contact with him, as he faded further out of reach from her caring grasp. The inevitable end that comes for all ALS patients was especially heart-wrenching in this case.

The next patient in this unlikely scenario was a home oxygen user. He was an uncompromising gentleman of sorts, who had advancing Chronic Obstructive Pulmonary Disease (COPD.) Cut from a rougher grade of cloth, he too was an outdoor enthusiast, often traveling with his truck and camper. His name wasn't Chester, but it should have been, so we will call him that for our purposes now. As an oxygen patient, Chester was one of those obstinate elderly types who was determined not only to keep on living life as normal, but to keep on smoking as normal also. And the mutually exclusive dynamic of the twin desires wasn't open to a lot of *patho-philosophical* discussion, either. He promised that he never smoked with his oxygen on, and I did my best to believe him.

Foremost again, since he was getting on in years and deteriorating in health, he wanted to continue his open road travels with his wife for as long as possible, and he needed more portability with his oxygen tanks. He didn't like altering his schedule and waiting for oxygen truck drivers to drop off another dozen portable tanks. Well, fortuitously at the time, the Invacare Company rolled out its Venture HomeFill Oxygen System, and he was the very first patient whom I switched over to a home refill unit. This system makes its own oxygen and safely pumps it into the portable, two thousand pounds per square inch cylinders. Do-it-yourself! There was no more waiting for the O_2 milkman to show up. Even better, he could pack the whole system into the back of his camper, and plug it into the 120-volt outlets provided at the campgrounds. Have pump, will travel: he was fully free now to move on down the road at will, and he and his wife certainly got their overland travel mileage in. From a manufacturer's marketing standpoint, he was probably the quintessential COPD patient type, who could really get the most out of this updated oxygen delivery technology. Except for the smoking!

Well, one routine morning I happened to be at Chester's house, performing some periodic purity checks on the oxygen concentrator in his bedroom. When I came back out, he was seated at the dining room table with his wife. He had a stack of papers in his hands that he was edge-tamping onto the tabletop. When he saw me, he made a subtle request.

"Mike. Get over here."

I walked over and he further offered cordially, "Have a seat."

As I was pulling out a chair he held up the small paper stack and said exuberantly, "I spent a lot of hours typing this story up. It is a really wild story about our honeymoon. And I want you to read it."

As I took my seat, I pensively looked over to the wife who was all smiles and then back to Chester again who was a combination of all smiles with an overlay of husky chest chuckles. My first thought was that as a licensed respiratory therapist on duty, I reserve the right to refuse to read wild honeymoon stories by anyone. *Especially when the wife is seated four feet away!*

I was privately uncertain of what to expect, but it looked like I had no choice in the matter at this point. So I took up the paper stack, and began reading to myself. (Chronologically, this reading occurred in January 2003, and the long-ago honeymoon had taken place forty-two years earlier, in 1961.) By the end of the first paragraph my eyes bugged out and I had to emote. It was breathtaking. I just couldn't believe it. Not verbatim, but the paragraph essentially read: "When my wife and I were young we spent a lot of time in the outdoors. In fact, when we decided to get married, we also decided that we would honeymoon far away from everybody. We planned to honeymoon for two whole weeks in the high wilderness. And we spent that time camping beside a high alpine lake in a small cabin that had a Trail Blazer's plaque on it...!"

As soon as I read that, I looked over and said, "Chester...you honeymooned in the Jewel Lakes in a remote cabin with a Trail Blazers plaque on it!?"

Chester responded impatiently, "Yeah, yeah. Keep going! Get to the *good stuff*!"

I said, "Chester, this *already is* the good stuff." Amazing coincidence at hand, I then quickly explained to them that I personally knew one of the original Trail Blazers who had actually assisted in the building of the cabin, and the mounting of that testimonial plaque. Wow! What were the chances of this? They of course were immediately interested in meeting this wonderful person (the builder of their rustic honeymoon suite!). And I further explained (without divulging too much personal health information) that he lived nearby, that he was a ventilator patient of mine, and that I would talk to his wife about, possibly, arranging a visit. As it later turned out, the wife (and the ALS patient) found it a moving and spectacular coincidence, and the two aged honeymooners did eventually pay a heartwarming visit to the stricken, magnificent Trail Blazer.

And with that serendipitous, preliminary resolution in place, we now return to the rest of the story—*Chester's good stuff*—the wild honeymoon! And it was indeed a wild honeymoon! You just can't make this stuff up. The post-nuptial escapades that occurred here were right out of Mr. Murphy's manual of unintended madness. What could go wrong would go wrong. And then some! And then some more! The best laid plans of mice and men are one thing, but special ops and airdrops over water are best left to military professionals.

The key honeymoon issue was how to survive for two whole weeks in such a high, remote territory. Given the long, precarious climb, it simply wasn't possible to carry two weeks' worth of provisions by backpack. Somehow, they needed to get many additional supplies up to the honeymoon lake, without involving any fellow hikers. So Chester came up with a grand plan to arrange an airdrop. He went to a flying service which existed back then called Bellevue Air (perhaps the precursor to Kenmore Air today), and presented them with a completed proposition. He already knew that the lakes were way too small for a float plane to land in, but maybe they could over-fly the lake and drop the supplies into the water, after which he would row out in a small rubber raft and retrieve them. And Chester had just the tactical devices needed to pull off the strategic mission: large, metal milk containers, three of them, almost waist high, with metal handles on each side. Perhaps you've seen the like at county fairs and so forth. The big cylindrical jugs tapered to a narrower neck and then flared back out again to a blunderbuss-type rim. Over the horn-like rim a large circular lid is secured by bending down the wire loops extending out around the edges of the lid.

 After fielding the details carefully, and after inspecting the empty jugs up close, the Bellevue Air pilot figured that this was a feasible proposition. The lids were air- and watertight, and the big jugs should easily float, after splashing into the water like a space capsule. Then the pilot devised a make-shift means to secure them in the plane, and a way quickly to release them when the time came. Finally, Chester and the pilot studied a graphic relief map of the lakes and the surrounding terrain. Given the rugged terrain, and the relatively small size of the lake, the pilot decided on a one-at-a-time, circle-around, three-drop strategy. He would make three passes over the high ridge, swoop down over the water, and drop each canister, trying to hit the center of the lake as squarely as possible. Further to distinguish the lake from the air, Chester would have his yellow, inflated raft tethered on the shoreline. When a canister hit the water, Chester could retrieve it while the plane climbed back up and around the ridge for the next drop.

Piece of cake. Angel cake even.

For something on the order of a hundred and fifty bucks, the great honeymoon airdrop was a go. Let's do this! Chester and his fiancé were excited, and the pilot thought it was a splendid aerial caper, particularly under the romantic circumstances. And since gravity did nearly all the work, what could possibly go wrong?

(Mr. Murphy taps his cigar and snickers, *oh, let me count the ways!*)

On schedule a week later, Chester and his new bride completed the initial, nine-mile climb by late on the first day. They camped in the Trail Blazer cabin that night, and were up early the next morning, preparing for the plane to arrive. Sun up, Chester inflated the folded rubber raft that he had ported up in his backpack and tethered it shore-side. The sky was perfectly clear, and it wasn't long before they heard the approaching drone of an aircraft, somewhere in the overhead distance. As they stood on a rock ledge beside the water, the ridge over which the plane was to come down was high up to their right. They watched; and, sure enough, the plane came over the crest and dived downward toward them. Still several hundred feet high, the plane then leveled off as it came over the approach end of the lake. The engine feathered (slowed to idle) and the right wing dipped. They immediately saw the first canister fall out of the craft, after which the pilot leveled the wings and throttled up the engine and sped ahead to make another go around.

The two watched anxiously as the earthbound canister vectored downward, but it also drifted dramatically to their left as it fell. Then it quickly became obvious that the canister was not going to hit the middle of the lake; it was going to carry beyond, and impact somewhere near the far end, to their left, where the water was very shallow. A wall of dense brush girded the shore on that side of the lake, with a thick stand of tall pine trees stationed immediately behind. The shallow water proved not to be a concern. The two winced and watched as the big jug slammed hard into the brush at the water's edge and bounced up high in the air, tumbling end over end like a football. It carried over the front row of pine trees and came down into the thick stand where they could hear the metal jug banging and whacking and slamming among the tree trunks like a pinball.

Ooops! It turned out that this first, ill-fated jug was the one containing all the dry goods: the flour, the sugar, the rice-a-roni, bags of bouillon, bags of chocolate milk powder, and so forth. The canister was severely dented and deformed, but miraculously the lid stayed on. But all the lid served to do was to preserve the mess inside. Later, sifting through the internal wreckage, they found that the bouillon powder bag and the chocolate powder had both exploded and co-mixed. A large box of rice-a-roni had likewise ruptured, and added its ingredients to the chocolate-bouillon concoction. Chester said that they actually tried a hot sample drink of the mixture, and it tasted pretty much as bizarre and disgusting as you might expect it to.

For the second pass, the airplane came over the ridge again, only this time it flew down much lower, and slower. Over the approach end of the water the engine cut quiet, the right wing dipped, and the next canister dropped out. The plane then accelerated away and the falling canister lit with a splash, out in the deep water directly in front of them. Perfect shot. Obviously it took one practice run to get this airdrop tactic right. Chester hopped in the raft and retrieved the canister pronto. This second jug was packed full with the extra bedding, clothing and jackets.

The third pass (as third times tend to be) was the charm. (Charming, like the glint of a gold tooth in Mr. Murphy's sinister grin.) The plane came down over the ridge for the final drop and this time it came extremely low, maybe fifteen to twenty feet above the water. Far back on the approach end, the engine feathered and the right wing dipped... and then it straightened up again...and then it dipped again... and then up again... something was wrong. The third canister was somehow stuck, and the pilot couldn't get it to release. As the newly-weds watched, perplexed, the plane throttled up loudly, as it sped up toward them. As the plane roared by out in front of them, the pilot in the door window gave them an up-thumb indication that he was going around to try it again.

The plane continued accelerating over the water, to about ninety miles an hour and then the pilot pulled the nose up, and, just as he did, the third canister somehow released on its own! Only now, it wasn't falling in a leisurely arc into the water. This canister was now a milk-jug missile going 90 miles an hour at a thirty-degree slant, headed right into the same zone that had demolished the first canister. It was now a Kamikaze torpedo on a mission to the netherworld.

The two grimacing newlyweds squatted down, palms on cheeks, almost unable to watch the energetic conclusion. Chester said that it all happened in less than two seconds. Like a torpedo, the jug hit the shallow water about twenty feet back from the water's edge. It skimmed ahead for about ten feet, sending back a huge rooster tail of water, and then, with a loud bang, the shoulder of the jug slammed into a rock ledge just beneath the surface and it came to an abrupt stop. It went from 90 miles an hour to 0 in about half a second. Instantly, faster than the human eye could comprehend it, the lid of the canister blew off and the entire contents of the jug shot-gunned out onto the shore side landscape, creating a huge debris field. In the blink of an eye—a splash, a bang and garbage splattered everywhere!

(For the infamous Mr. Murphy, it was now a glorious moment to twiddle his cigar, to shake his booty, and to do the moonwalk, all at the same time.)

For the disheartened newlyweds, however, it was now a morbid moment to begin the grim task of searching for surviving meals. They needed every bit of the food to survive the two weeks as planned, and this was the most important canister. It had all the major food staples in it: the fresh meats, canned meat, bread, cheese, vegetables and the like. They anxiously made their way around the lake through the brush, to try to salvage whatever they could.

Some food items were easier to recoup than others. As it turned out, packed right on top in the canister, and the first item to leave the cannon barrel, was five pounds of sliced bacon, wrapped in loose butcher paper. The bacon slices had shredded apart through the air, and were now hanging in festoons everywhere. Dangling bacon slices littered everything from the shoreline brush to the high branches of the pine trees.

Slice by slice, they focused on retrieving all the low-hanging bacon first. Along the way, they came across a couple of limp, hanging bags of Wonderbread, skewered on bush sticks. Much of the bread was missing, but they found many individual slices and pieces scattered deeper back into the branches. They gathered up as many of the remaining bread clumps as they could. In digging for the more visible white bread pieces they happened upon several stray potatoes and broken carrots. Behind the brush, they found what became a permanent curiosity. It had slammed hard into one of the forward tree trunks and it now lay empty on the ground. It was the exploded blue can of the 3-pound Denmark ham that was earmarked for at least two or three meals. The can was crushed, the lid splayed open, with only slight remnants of packing jelly on the inside surface. The ham itself was nowhere to be found. Even after several return trips in the ensuing days, they couldn't locate a single piece of it. They figured that here had to be some large, salvageable chunks of ham lying around in the pine needles somewhere in the vicinity. The salty ham would keep for many days and it would be easy to just to wash it off and to fry it up. But no such luck. Those canned hams do have a high water content, and Chester suggested humorously that maybe the whole thing had just vaporized on impact!

Having retrieved all that they could within ground level reach, they then shifted focus to the bacon slices hanging high in the pine branches overhead. Strewn helter-skelter like decorations on the evergreens, the bacon slices hung there like some kind of "Bubba's Christmas tree tinsel."

They searched the deadfall for old limbs, and using a hunting knife, they whittled and fashioned some long sticks with a branch hook at the end. They moved along the tree line, reaching up and lifting down the remaining bacon slices one by one. Along the way, another curiosity presented itself. Attached to one of the tree trunks was what appeared to be a toadstool. Most of us have seen toadstools before, clinging to tree trunks like a half-moon section of giant mushroom. This toadstool fitted the general half-moon profile, but it wasn't gray-white in color like the traditional species. This one was bright orange. Upon closer inspection it turned out not to be a toadstool at all, but a deformed, two-pound block of cheddar cheese that had pasted itself to the pine tree trunk. Using his belt knife, Chester gently pried the cheese-stool away from the tree. Beneath the cheese were trickles of pinesap on the bark, and some of the sticky sap and bark bits had been impregnated into the cheese. But according to Chester and his wife, when sliced up, the evergreen accents actually added a "foresty" taste to the cheese that wasn't that bad at all. Perhaps it was the one unintended pleasantry of the otherwise unintended disaster that had begun their honeymoon stay.

But in the end, owing to an inspiring and glorious dynamic, the honeymooners recovered well.

In the final analysis, as the ever-puckish Mr. Murphy would have it, the only canister that made a safe splash down was the one containing the extra bedding and clothes. The two other critical food canisters, of course, took a Newtonian beating of devastating proportions. But, even with the laws of physics at his insidious disposal, Mr. Murphy ultimately failed in his vile attempt to quash the honeymoon plan. Granted, he had severely depleted the honeymooner's primary food stock, but in the high and mighty grandeur writ large across this magnificent alpine landscape, his misuse of the laws of physics proved no match for the indomitable spirit of the ALS patient and his beloved Trail Blazer's Club.

The final perspective that brings this incredible coincidence to full-circle fruition, is that, despite the loss of many meals in the aerial caper, the honeymooners were still able to complete their full two-week stay by filling in all the gaps in their shattered menu with, of all things...trout from the lake!

Thankfully, there were trout aplenty. And who had first put those trout there a few years prior? None other than the wonderful ALS patient and his Trail Blazer compatriots.

The happy honeymooners didn't just owe the Trail Blazers a debt of gratitude for the cabin accommodations alone, but for all the trip-saving meals as well. Nourished and sheltered, they were in good hands the whole time. And who could have ever predicted that trout, precariously stocked in a faraway lake, would someday rescue a troubled honeymoon from disaster? But it did. Somehow, wonderfully, it was all meant to be. And I am ever so thankful that I was able to learn about the whole coincidental and uplifting episode and to pass it on to others. Not only is life a miracle in itself, but it can also be inexplicably amazing after the fact.

The Tragedy of Tripping Hazards and Fatal Falls in the Home

All homecare medical professionals (respiratory therapists, nurses, occupational therapists, physical therapists, social workers, etc.) who perform in-home patient care are required to instruct patients on the dangers of tripping hazards in the home. In 2008 the Joint Commission* made Fall Prevention Awareness a mandatory part of hospital employee and in-home patient education. Currently, thousands of elderly patients die in their homes due to preventable falling accidents. And this statistical morbidity is compounded by fall victims who could have survived had they been rescued in time. The physical or technical inability to call for timely help is a problem within the problem for many vulnerable elderly people. Thankfully, remote alert devices are increasingly being utilized. But ultimately, by way of routine medical contact, Fall Prevention Education needs to be relentlessly inculcated and practiced, because, as shown in following National Safety Council brief, the statistics are still much too ugly.

According to the National Safety Council, falls are one of the leading causes of unintentional injuries in the United States, accounting for approximately 8.9 million visits to the emergency department. Falls are the second most frequent cause of unintentional death in homes and communities, resulting in more than twenty-five thousand fatalities in 2009. The risk of falling, and fall-related problems, rises with age, and is a serious issue in homes and communities (2011 NSC Injury Facts).[1]

Unfortunately, I experienced this domestic menace at first hand, very early in my respiratory therapy career. My first (and by far still worst) patient-care encounter with a fatal falling incident occurred in the Philadelphia area in 1978. At the time, I was employed full time at the Sacred Heart Hospital in Norristown, PA, and I also worked part-time for an upstart Homecare Company called Respiratory Rentals, from the Plymouth Meeting area. In those years, the ubiquitous Continuous Positive Airway Pressure machine (CPAP) hadn't even been invented yet, and most respiratory homecare centered on in-home Intermittent Positive Pressure Breathing machines (IPPB), particularly the venerable Bennett AP-5. I serviced a collection of fifteen IPPB patients, scattered out in the Northwest sector beyond Philadelphia in the Montgomery and Bucks county regions. I was required personally to check their equipment and medicines once a month, or more often if they called and requested assistance.

Over all, it was a pleasant and scenic outing, when taking care of most of these patients. The Penn Dutch countryside rolling out beyond Philadelphia is a beautiful region, and I drove through a lot of "postcard" scenery in my rounds. The natural rolling green pastures and tree groves were adorned with man-made silos, farmhouses and painted barns. Amish horse-drawn buggies added their vintage charm to the scenery, and making for my own favorite post-card aesthetic, all along the rural roadways, *real pheasants on fence posts* added a colorful punctuation to the foreground. Finally, the farmland landscape was, hither and yon, adorned with small, rustic stone bridges that spanned gentle flowing creeks, antiquated remnants from much simpler and bygone times.

But alternatively, modern socio-economic factors being what they are, there were also some difficult regions to travel as well. A handful of my patients lived in some downtrodden urban areas that stretched from Manyunk to Bridgeport and up to Southwest Norristown. One unfortunate patient lived in a tiny multiplex, along the railroad tracks, where the living-room sliding glass door was literally twenty feet removed from passing trains. The roar of a passing train would suffocate the entire house; you couldn't hear the TV or talk to the person sitting next to you. It was disheartening to experience some of the difficult living conditions that some elderly folks had to endure.

But the tragic falling incident itself involved an elderly, wiry, seventy-year-old Italian man, whom we will call Vinny. He lived in a small apartment above a run-down urban Moose Lodge. The relatively sparse patrons entered the lodge in front from a dirt parking lot, while Vinny, the apartment dweller, scaled some wrought iron steps on the side of the building that led to the upper-story doorway. I had climbed the rusty welded staircase many times, and the old man would dutifully leave the screen door and inner door unlocked when he knew I was coming. On my last visit, about two weeks prior to the tragedy, I went up the steps and the inner door was already open. I rapped at the screen door, but got no answer. I opened the screen door and peeked my head inside and called his name. Still no answer. I went into the small living room and called his name, and again no answer. The bathroom door was open and unoccupied, so I moved on past to the kitchen. In the back of the kitchen was an open door that I wasn't familiar with. Peering beyond the doorway I saw a steep set of wooden stairs that led downward into a gloomy, almost dark storage area. I walked down the steps slowly and found myself standing in among rows of shelves containing boxes of canned soup, and other bulk restaurant supplies. Ahead was a lighted glow, so I moved toward it and I emerged into the cook's work area behind the grill, and there I found Vinny. He was seated on a barstool with a towel draped around his neck. Standing behind him was the apparent barber, with a pair of scissors and an electric razor. Vinny acknowledged me and I introduced myself, and the jovial barber-cook paused, and without relocating his feet, set the razor down and reached back to the grill and flipped a couple hamburgers and then resumed trimming Vinny's hair. This was an interesting work arrangement to say the least. The Moose Lodge Grill and Barbershop? Then the combo grill-master and hair-stylist asked if I wanted a hamburger myself, and I politely declined. The proximity of the two interactive enterprises had an unappetizing ambiance to it. I was only twenty-two years old at the time, and I learned early on that you will see a lot of strange human endeavor in respiratory home care that you may not ever see otherwise. (Or even want to see.)

Unfortunately, you also inevitably experience the loss of patients to whom you have grown personally close. A couple weeks later I came to work at Sacred Heart in the morning and right away noticed Vinny's name on the Critical Care Cardex. He had been admitted comatose through the Emergency Room the evening before. He was now on a ventilator. He had slipped and fallen in his kitchen three days earlier, had struck his left forehead full on to the edge of the kitchen counter, and had cracked his skull. No one had missed him for the three days that he had lain helpless on the floor, not even the Moose Lodge friends just one floor below. I went to his ICU room to check on him. No longer comatose, he was deeply groggy, but at least cognizant of who I was. However, the grotesque swelling of the whole left side of his head was of a magnitude I hadn't seen before. Untreated for days, the swollen edematous mass on the left face had its own bulging eyeball that was three times the size of the unaffected one. With no attempt to be gratuitous, just to be objective about the tragic injury, it was as if an oversize purple alien head was morphing out of a normal human head. It was a godawful injury to behold. And it wasn't a horrific head trauma sustained from crashing through the windshield of a car, nor from a heavy equipment construction accident, but from just a quick fall within the otherwise safe confines of home. To have sustained such an equivalent level of massive head trauma at home would seem impossible, but tragically, it is not so. Consequently, one can never be too careful about falling in the home, and furthermore diligent in teaching our elderly patients especially to be routinely aware of the many potential tripping and falling hazards in the home. (See reference list)

Vinny passed away within the next few days, a tragic example of an all too common occurrence in the home. Hopefully his mournful retrospective will provide both cause and inspiration for all clinicians and family members to take home safety and fall prevention very seriously.

* Joint Commission on Healthcare Accreditation. (Accredits and certifies more than 20,500 health care organizations and programs in the United States.)

References

1. Slips, Trips and Falls Prevention, Fact Sheets & Statistics. (2014). Retrieved July 6, 2014, from http://www.nsc.org/safety_home/HomeandRecreationalSafety/Falls/Pages/Falls.aspx

Trading Places. In the Morgue
An Instructive Lesson in Communicating with the Dead

Linguistically, the verbal phrase *communicating with the dead* has at least a couple of dramatically different meanings. The more straightforward meaning of the participial phrase would bring to mind a séance, wherein, through a medium, participants achieve a heightened state of mind, in which communications from the dead can be heard or exchanged. From the standpoint of grammar, this highly paranormal interaction constitutes the *objective sense* of the phrase: In a séance, ostensibly, the dead and the living are objectively communicating to each other.

Now, if you think that that is crazy or spooky or worse, the illustration of the *subjective sense* (or *gerund* form) of the verbal phrase will really give you the creeps. Unavoidably, this will entail some unsettling and even gory scenarios to contemplate. For instance, in the same manner that one can *communicate with a puppet* (to an audience), if one were, instead, to substitute a real corpse for the puppet on stage, and, for example, to manipulate one of the hands and tell a story in sign language, one would be—however gruesomely—*communicating with the dead*. In other words, one is subjectively utilizing a dead body to communicate a message to others. Grotesque as that may sound hypothetically, there are actually some macabre, real-world spin-offs on this necro-communicational theme. Without dwelling too deeply upon the darker underworld of humanity, the mob has been well known to communicate with the dead, sometimes disfiguring the cadavers in creatively morbid ways to add special emphasis to the message. But to segue back to the nobler side of hospital work and respiratory care, this subjective fashion of communicating with the dead was actually brought to bear one time in a hospital, circa 1977. And, as expected, the tactic had an enormous impact on the recipient of the message, especially since the messenger wasn't quite as dead as he was alleged to be.

    This remedial and justifiably punitive caper took place at a hospital in eastern Pennsylvania (although eastern Transylvania would be more fitting.) The antagonist in this *employee-relations* scenario was a hospital orderly, who was about as cocky and cornball a person as one would care to meet. He was a well-built, blond, tanned, gum-chomping, Jersey-shore beach-boy type, who so loved to dig his own act that you'd swear, if he could clone himself—he'd marry himself. (A real man for the biotechnological age.) Anyway, if this self-centered schmuck wasn't grandstanding for the nurses, and palavering and boasting about off color exploits, he'd be off indulging in his notorious role as a prankster, pulling pesky tricks on other hospital staff members and just being an all-around nuisance. Call it a personality clash, or what have you, this puckish lout just had an irritating quality about him that radiated through any vicinity he occupied, and made fellow occupants uncomfortable. But he did finally receive his belated comeuppance one night, when he took his brazen silliness more than just a little too far.

One night, about ten o'clock, when most hospital patients were asleep, and the evening work shift was winding down, the prankster orderly quietly slipped into a vacant room, down the hall from the nurses' station and pressed the bedside call button.

At that moment (as the orderly had plotted) there was only one, younger nurse-in-training at the station. She responded promptly to the call light and headed down the hall toward the room. As she approached the doorway, she paused, puzzled. She had thought that this was a vacant room, but obviously she must be mistaken. She leaned her head into the dark doorway, but couldn't see anybody. She moved inside, a step or two more, and suddenly a hand from behind the bedside curtain closed over her mouth and face! Her scream was completely muffled by the thick palm, and the orderly promptly spun her out into the lighted hallway and cackled—"Surprise!"

Needless to say, it was not funny. It was not funny at all. And sensing that he might have really gone over the top this time, the orderly made a quick apology and then scooted out to attend to work elsewhere in the facility. (Parenthetical caveat: this was many years ago. Interpersonal charades were much more loosey-goosey back then. Do not even think of attempting this kind of bodily antic in today's work place environment. Workplace violence and sexual harassment rules will ensure a rapid pink slip ticket to the unemployment line. Ultimately, for all brazen, macho knuckleheads out there—keep your hands to yourself!) But back to the scene. Too flustered even to reprimand the imbecile, the student nurse immediately returned to the station, where she sat frightened, trying to compose herself.

Shortly thereafter, two respiratory therapists named Steve and Tom came onto the station. Steve was in his early thirties, sporting wire-rimmed spectacles, a slender, outdoorsy, Air Force Vietnam veteran. Disciplined, educated, he hated all pranksters in general—the orderly's guts in particular. Tom was a big farm boy of sorts, mid-twenties, a tall, strong, college tight end (University of Tulsa). He occasionally smiled, rarely budged on a topic, and seemed imposing; but he was actually a sedate, muscular teddy bear in his own taciturn kind of way.

Upon learning of this latest, pathetic prank, Steve and Tom resolved to pluck this miserable turkey in his own barnyard once and for all. Enough was enough. The two of them quickly developed a plan and then notified all the nurses in that wing as to what was going down and how they could assist with the choreography.

Tom and Steve wheeled in a crash cart and an array of resuscitation equipment, and set it up in a vacant room at the very end of the hall. Big Tom undressed, put on a patient gown and got into bed. Blankets were piled loosely over his head and large frame, in such a manner that he could breathe incognito. A collection of emergency packs, oxygen supplies and defibrillator equipment was scattered about the bedside to simulate that a real medical emergency had taken place. Meanwhile the nurses quickly made a phony patient

I.D. card, along with some bogus documents and chart forms.

Ultimately, whenever a death in the hospital occurred, it was the orderly's task to process the identification paper work, and to transport the body to the morgue. All things set and ready, they promptly put in a call for the doomsday dude.

When the orderly arrived at the room, Steve was somberly repackaging some equipment while a couple of teary-eyed nurses stood at the foot of the bed, quietly consoling each other.

Chewing his gum slowly, the orderly whispered at Steve, "What happened?"

Steve rolled his eyes and then shook his head as if too exasperated to talk. Then he said, in a tone of restrained anger, "A real screw-up! A medication error or something! The nurses killed this guy! I'll tell you, someone's butt is going to hang in hell for this!"

The orderly's eyes swelled, as his jaw hung in mid chomp. Then he asked, "Which nurse did it?"

"Doesn't matter," Steve asserted. "Just listen up. There is a special pathologist flying in from New York tonight to handle the case. The medical director said to take the body to the morgue and not to disturb anything; not the blankets, the pillows, nothing. It could all be state's evidence. Just tag the toe and park him downstairs."

Partly spooked, but mostly intrigued, the orderly mashed his gum openly with his big teeth. "Heavy-duty screw-up, huh?" he sighed introspectively, grinning and chewing and shaking his head.

Steve nodded disgustedly, not sharing the orderly's insipid enthusiasm for the tragedy. Then he quickly stepped away, before he started grinning himself.

For the next several minutes, the orderly made the scene, standing there in the thick of things, foot propped on the bed frame, doing the paperwork on his knee, scribbling importantly, as still-another somber-faced nurse brought his morbid majesty some more bogus forms to autograph. Yes, indeed, wouldn't the ladies at the bar be impressed with this new episode: catastrophic medical errors, nurses in deep trouble, special inquests pending, dead bodies to the morgue...all in a day's work, chomp, chomp.

After the ceremonial toe-tagging had been completed, the now stern-faced orderly took center stage on parade, as he wheeled the blanketed body out into the hallway and rolled it down the corridor to the elevator. A small coterie of mourners followed to give their send-off, and, when the elevator doors closed, the orderly was ostensibly on his own.

At the basement level, he pushed the body out of the elevator and down the long, dreary, cinderblock hallway to the infamous room number *thirteen,* a common designation for the morgue in many Christian hospitals. (In fact, the overhead audio announcement of "conference in room thirteen" is often the surreptitious call for those who need to know that an autopsy is soon to begin.) At the morgue entrance, he unlocked the big double doors, wheeled the bed inside, and parked it parallel to the shiny, stainless steel autopsy table. Opposite the body, a short distance away, were a small office desk and phone, up next to the wall. The orderly turned around, moved to the desk, and began to open the thick, gilded logbook of no return. It was an eerie ledger, containing the accumulated, mortal names of those bygone souls who had terminally checked out, never to check back in.

He thought.

Ever so slowly, Tom peeled the blanket away from his head, and off his body, as the orderly scribbled, oblivious. He bent his knees, and carefully brought his feet over the edge of the mattress. He quietly drew a huge breath and then—with the explosive burst of a football player coming off the line of scrimmage—he shattered the silence and launched out with a loud, guttural scream and bear hugged the orderly from behind. Tom manhandled him up, and shook him around like a big rag doll, still howling like a mad werewolf. Then he let him down and released him, spinning him around to the side as the orderly had done to the nurse earlier.

"Surprise!" Tom bellowed into his face.

Stunned, the orderly didn't respond. His face was expressionless and faded in color. He leaned back and bumped into the wall adjacent to the desk, and then he slid down to his rump on the floor. He seemed to stare blankly, but calmly.

Standing above, Tom leaned down into his face again and repeated, "Hey guy! Surprise!"

Still again, gawking like a zombie on Propofol, the orderly made no response. And then, as Tom watched, the orderly's face tilted backward and his eyes rolled to the top of his head! Almost a sure indication that his heart had stopped beating! All of a sudden, it appeared that the two of them had actually traded places in the morgue, only, in this instance, the orderly wasn't faking it!

Now Tom got scared, real scared. He jumped down and grabbed the orderly's wrist. No pulse! He felt his neck. No pulse! He peppered his cheeks desperately a few times and pleaded, "Wake up! Wake up!"

But there was still no response. He looked up at the desk phone. Then back to the orderly. His drooping face was the color of bread dough. This guy had seriously arrested! There was only one thing to do: pick up the phone, dial the access code to the intercom, and announce a Code Blue emergency and call the resuscitation team to the morgue! Code Blue! Morgue?! And oh, how that medically incongruent announcement was going to prickle every nape in the building, as well as give the hospital administrators something seriously to investigate the next morning.

Tom knew the drill: grab the phone, make the call, start Cardio-Pulmonary-Resuscitation. Just as Tom grabbed the phone, the orderly groaned and began to come out of his shock. Relieved, Tom put the phone down, sat back into the office chair, and continued to observe the orderly, seated on the floor in front of him. For the first time, Tom noticed that the orderly's white polyester pants were profusely damp in front. It was a fitting, if not humbling touch, under the circumstances. Hopefully, that was the extent of it. (In fact, given the modern impetus for evidenced-based protocols, overwhelming evidence abounded here that it was indeed clinically feasible to "frighten the urine" out of some one.)

Still gaunt and staring, all of sudden the orderly began panting rhythmically, as if he had just remembered that he hadn't been breathing for a while and needed to catch up. Then his eyes regained some cognizance and he started to look around, while copious trickles of sweat ran down his cheeks.

Still gathering and reassembling his wits, the stricken orderly studied his surroundings for a while longer, until the full picture finally congealed in his head. Then he looked up to Tom and protested timidly: "That ain't funny, man."

Big Tom grinned. Message delivered. Lesson learned.

Rookie Mistakes in Respiratory Care

For all nursing and allied health professionals, the collective, working modus operandi of *quality patient care* is governed by a combination of *The Five Rights*, coupled with interactive *collaboration* between all parties directly involved in the care of each patient.

Like most important dynamics in life, co-ordinating maximal patient cared is much easier said than done.

The Five Rights of patient care are—to treat the *right* patient, with the *right* medicine, at the *right* time, in the *right* dosage, by the *right* route. As originally written, these fundamental Five Rights apply more specifically to bedside nursing procedures, but the larger concept extends to all allied health practitioners from RT, PT, OT, Radiology, Nutritionist, social workers, etc. We must all strive to treat the right patient with the right therapy, at the right time, in the right manner and, at the same time, try to coordinate and schedule said therapies with each other to achieve maximum benefit for the patient. (Again, easier said than done.) For instance, an asthmatic patient with a recent knee replacement surgery is going to PT for exercise routines. Having the RT department schedule the QID bronchodilator treatment prior to the exercise appointment would be beneficial, if it can be arranged. But someone needs to be aware of the bigger picture, in order to have that beneficial sequence arranged and enacted.

From a hierarchical standpoint, the best way to view patient care is from the innermost orbit of nursing care. Each patient has an assigned nurse who is ultimately responsible for his or her care plan and daily activities. All other allied health professionals orbit around the nursing component, and must interact accordingly. If there is any desire or doubt about any aspect of the patient's care, the attending nurse must be appraised and included in the discussion. And then, so too, the patient's doctor, as needed. The above asthmatic scenario would be a case in point. But even something as innocuous as a patient's having asked a therapist for a glass of water may need to be considered. Maybe the patient is NPO (nothing by mouth) pending an upcoming procedure. One never knows, until things are checked out. But ultimately, you have to train yourself to be cognizant enough even to think to check these kinds of things out. (Ergo, easier said than done.) Ultimately, experience is the best teacher. And sometimes, inevitably, experience hurts.

With that said and done, we address the topic of patient care mistakes. We all make mistakes in our chosen professions, especially early on, and even more so early on as a student. All nursing and allied health professions require extensive observation and mentorship from clinical preceptors, in order to become proficient, and to gain the confidence eventually to become an independent, licensed practitioner. And even then, continuing education and re-certification becomes a career-long process. But we all start working at some point, and I made two mistakes in my working student years that were very instructive at the time. The practice in years past was more lenient toward students. While still in school, unlicensed RT students could actually get hired by a hospital to perform, independently, certain (lower-level) procedures, while still not being allowed to perform certain higher-level ones. These were designated "student gopher" positions, and they were a great opportunity both to earn money and to get clinical experience at the same time. Since they were paid hours, they didn't count as clinical hours for school, but they were just as instructive. For instance, myself, as a student, part way through the RT program in Tacoma in 1976, I got a student gopher position at St. Joseph's Hospital, making $2.90 an hour. I was cleared to do IPPB treatments, incentive spirometry and chest physical therapy, but I was not allowed to perform ventilator checks, nor to draw arterial blood samples, nor to perform CPR with the Code Four team. And if an ER emergency or Code Four happened, and the full time therapists were tied up with it, as the designated gopher, I took over their routine patient work for the time being. After all, that's what student gophers are for.

My first major mistake was right out of the Five Rs. The First R in fact! The right patient! Believe me, you hate it when this happens. My only consolation is that, thankfully, I was just a student RT at the time, and not a practicing surgeon! (We've all heard those outrageous stories before.) Anyway, it was after eleven p.m., at the end of the three to eleven shift, and I was finishing report with the nightshift, and was about to go home. Then a call came up from the ER to do an IPPB treatment on a patient in room E-4. Since I was the solitary gopher, and since the shift wasn't technically over for another fifteen minutes, all eyes shifted to me. I knew my place in the pecking order, and so did they. To my colleagues' credit, they weren't about to interfere with my opportunity further to enrich my educational experience.

Now, at that point in time, I had taken one orientation trip through the Emergency Room, but had never worked there, as I wasn't cleared for most emergencies yet. But this was a routine IPPB (breathing) treatment, so it was OK.

Ten floors below, there were two (authorized-only) back doors to the ER from the hallway, so I took the nearest one, remembering the room number, E-4. Ahead along the wall, to my left, were six rooms, all of them dark and unoccupied except for the brightly-lit room #4. It was a no brainer. I immediately wheeled in my trusty Bird Mark 7 IPPB unit on its wheel stand, and met an elderly gentleman laying on a gurney. His right leg was bandaged and his knee was elevated on a roll pad. In my well-practiced, chipper style, I introduced myself as the respiratory therapist and then briefly explained what the machine and the treatment were designed to do, and that I would need to take his pulse and listen to his breath sounds.

Scowling, he asked, tersely, "What is this all about?"

I paused in the application of my stethoscope and re-explained that the doctor had ordered a bronchodilator treatment for him to reduce bronchoconstriction and to ease the work of breathing. "This machine and mouth piece will make a medicine mist that you will breathe in and then exhale back out the through the mouthpiece."

He countered, "Look, I'm breathing fine. I just want to get out of here. I've been here too long already."

I assured him that this would not take more than fifteen minutes, and he shook his head, annoyed, but reluctantly went along with it. After the pre-assessment I handed him the green tubing and nebulizer assembly and had him take his first breath on the IPPB unit. After a few breaths he immediately groused, "what is this stuff? It tastes awful!"

"It is a medication called Bronkosol," I told him...and that was about as far as I got.

A nurse appeared at the doorway and addressed me forthrightly. "What are you doing? This is the wrong patient for the IPPB treatment!"

The patient looked at me and crabbed, "Oh, for crying out loud, get this thing away from me." And he flung the nebulizer tubing back at me.

Flustered, embarrassed and immediately sick to my stomach, I apologized to the patient, and he didn't want to hear about it. The nurse had me gather up my equipment, and she escorted me out to the station where she further explained to me that the proper room was E-4, not T-4. The E-side rooms were Exam rooms, and the T-side rooms were Treatment rooms. And why didn't I already know that? And why didn't I check in with her first, to begin with? Crestfallen, I didn't have an answer for either, but there was still an asthmatic patient to be cared for so she directed me pronto to the proper room to get that done. I tried to keep my spirits up as I gave the IPPB treatment to the wheezing lady in room E-4.

After I finished the treatment, the ER nurse had me sit down at her station desk, and fill out and sign an incident report. It took about half an hour to complete the long form, and I was nauseated the whole time. It was the longest thirty minutes of my life, as I sat there in the open, like some penitent delinquent, dutifully filling in the blanks while other on-duty nurses, doctors and EMT personnel circulated around me. I felt so lowly and unworthy—like a fungus in the medical fruit salad—a dorky dilettante who had just contaminated the highly professional environment at large.

Downtrodden, I eventually skulked back up to the twelfth floor to report out to the night shift, and (God bless her) Joanne assured me that the misery I was feeling would pass on in due time. It wasn't a terminal ventilator mistake, or an accidental Isuprel overdose. Ultimately, you failed to check in with the nurse first, and get your bearings. It was a well-meaning, but over-eager rookie misstep. You got in a hurry, and you didn't fully check things out, and it bit you. And it hurts. And you'll learn from it. And I did.

I thought.

Sometimes you can get into patient care trouble without even realizing it in the least. The old adage that no good deed ever goes unpunished is especially apt here. It was about six months later; I had transferred my "student gopher" credential from St. Joseph's Hospital across town to Lakewood General Hospital. I was further along in my studies, and was now cleared to perform all aspects and procedures of respiratory care. Plus, the RT department at

Lakewood General was also tasked with doing electrocardiograms. Although it was a much smaller community hospital, LGH operated a true cardiopulmonary department. And I found that interesting and challenging. (I also found that LGH paid student gophers three dollars fifty an hour instead of two dollars ninety. Not much of a difference, seemingly? It is almost a twenty-one per cent raise! Do the math.)

But I digress. My second rookie mistake was so casually inadvertent that, afterward, it propelled me to an even deeper level of "check with the nurse first." (Don't spit into the wind, never leave your wingman, and always check with the nurse first—especially if the patient has any signs of dementia.) It was a cold, rainy April evening, at about seven p.m. I was called to do an electrocardiogram on a patient in a room on One West, in bed number two. These were twin-bed rooms and bed number one was closest to the door, and bed number two against the window. I wheeled the EKG machine into the room, parked it at the foot of bed number two, and identified the patient as the one needing the EKG.

Before I got started, the elderly man sitting up in bed #1 said to me, "Sonny, could you do me a favor and get my shoes for me?" I paused and went over to the other side of his bed to get his shoes, and he further asked me to get his coat out of the closet. He said he was cold. So I reached in and retrieved that too. He told me that he had a bad back and couldn't reach down very well and could I put the shoes on for him. The man already had black socks on; otherwise he was wearing just a hospital gown, and he also had a urinary catheter bag hanging on the lower bed frame. I knelt down and put his hard black loafers on and then draped his coat over his shoulders. That seemed to make him comfy, and he thanked me for my help and I then pulled the bedside curtain between them to perform the EKG on his neighbor.

Afterward I returned to the RT department and finished cutting and pasting the long EKG strip into its individual twelve-lead placements on the finished sheet, and then I put the sheet in the box down the hall, to be read by the cardiologist at a later time. (The old-fashioned way! Today twelve-lead EKGs are completed, interpreted, and printed within seconds, literally before you can get the wires removed from the patient's limbs and chest.)

I then went off to do my therapy rounds on the upper floor, and it was about two hours later when I returned to the department that my cohort Joe Morton informed me that he just got a call and I needed to go and speak with the nursing supervisor on One West. They were very upset with me!

I was stymied. Upset with me? Upset about what?

Joe said, "Something about a patient you dealt with. I guess the police had to get involved. You need to go talk with them"

"The *police?*" I yelped aghast. At this point, I was about as flabbergasted as I'd ever been on the job. What could this possibly be about? Spooked, I made a beeline to the nursing supervisor, and she was quick to scold me about sending a dementia patient out into the night. "And why would I do that?"

Wonked, I asked her for more detail, I didn't understand, I had no clue what was going on here. She explained that "Mr. So-and-so said that you put his shoes and coat on him and then told him that he could go home now. So he picked up his catheter bag and hung it on his finger and walked out the front entrance into the pouring rain."

Holy moly! I hurried to explain that I did put his shoes and coat on him, but only as a bedside favor, to keep him warm at his request. I did not in any way instruct him, nor insinuate that he was free to leave. Obviously I have no authority to discharge any patient.

She accepted my explanation, and further detailed that the poor rain-soaked man had ended up on someone's front porch, about a half mile down the road. The startled family opened their front door to find him standing there, holding his catheter bag, completely drenched, in his overcoat and hospital gown and bare legs with black loafers. The family called the police, and they eventually returned him to the hospital. What a bizarre sequence; thankfully, the old man wasn't injured in the process.

Although not technically implicated in anything, I was part of the sequence that enabled him to leave, so I still had to complete another long, explanatory incident report about the affair, and what course of correction would be necessary to prevent such an incident in the future. Sometimes you are not really sure what ameliorative actions to suggest, but you can never be too careful about assessing a patient's current condition, needs and intentions, and that includes ALL PATIENTS, not just the ones you are working with. You must expand your field of clinical vision and responsibility. And certainly, for the protection of any patients at risk for episodes of dementia, health care workers need especially to attune their concerns and watchfulness.

In the end, the current mantra of treating all mistakes as an opportunity for improvement is well directed. In deference to Vince Lombardi, in the medical world especially, learning from mistakes isn't everything, it is the only thing.

Medical Incompetence and Opportunities for Improvement... or Skipping Town?

Medical incompetence can have innumerable forms and manifestations. But in spite of that, all of the forms and manifestations have one thing in common. Incompetence. Quite frankly, some clinician is either performing a procedure that they are not qualified to do, or they are qualified, but make a careless error at the time due to distraction, inattention, or lack of recent practice. Exactly where incompetence becomes malpractice is an issue, which I will leave to the lawyers. Not every clumsy goof in a medical procedure leads to significant pain and suffering and an impending lawsuit. And perhaps, sometimes, a simple apology can rectify the situation entirely. In every case, though, mild or serious, workable solutions have emerged in terms like, "opportunity for improvement," and "teachable moment," and the like. In every case, we must endeavor to learn from all medical mistakes. Especially the serious ones.

    Only once in my long respiratory therapy career did I witness frank incompetence by a doctor that certainly encroached on the border of malpractice, if not crossing it outright. Now stereotypically, a lot of lay people have this vision of malpractice as being perpetrated by some egotistical jerk doctor who is overbearing and careless and indifferent to a patient's pain. Maybe it's always like that on television, but certainly not so here. This is the case of a very genteel, attentive and highly intelligent doctor who simply should not have been performing the invasive procedure at hand. He obviously wasn't trained for it. The abbreviated procedure resulted in the traumatizing of a patient's throat and vocal cords, and, ultimately, the removal of the physician's temporary privileges, pending a medical board review. In the days leading up to the board review, the soft-spoken, genteel doctor gently skipped town.

(As a parenthetical aside, regarding those hypothetical, egotistical jerk doctors, they do exist, in very small numbers. And there are times when hospital staff would like to see them skip town too. But not infrequently, they can also be highly competent jerks, so you are stuck with them.)

Note: *Absolutely all of the highly competent Tacoma-area Pulmonologists are thoroughly exempt from the previous sentiment.*

This episode of medical incompetence emerged at Puget Sound Hospital in Tacoma, WA. circa 1984. The new Texas Corporation, that had purchased and remodeled the hospital facility (two years earlier) had also built the Soundview Clinic facilities across the street. To fill the new clinic offices, they recruited many doctors from around the country and from the military services, and encouraged them to bring their practices to Tacoma and to take advantage of discounted leasing rates. Many wonderful young doctors came to town then, and many are still practicing in the area today. (Of parenthetical note, one of the doctors was a noted pioneer of laparoscopic gall bladder surgery. It was yet another prestigious coup for little old Puget Sound Hospital.)

Another newly recruited doctor at the time was a soft spoken, diminutive man from the East Coast. He was something on the order of an internal medicine / family practice doctor. He was so new that all his paperwork had not been processed yet, but he had been granted temporary privileges by the hospital medical board. He paid a friendly visit to our respiratory therapy department on his own behalf, and he had many questions about our respiratory equipment and procedures. He mentioned that, as part of his new family practice, he was going to be performing fiber-optic bronchoscopy on his patients in the near future.

Now, the Tacoma area (let me assure you) has never wanted for superlative pulmonologists. In fact, back then especially, if Tacoma had been deemed to be the pulmonology capital of the world, it wouldn't have surprised me. In fact, I would probably posit further, "do pulmonologists exist on Mars or Jupiter?" Obviously not, of course, so that would make Tacoma at least the pulmonology capital of the solar system. But I do have a hometown bias to be sure.

Anyway, as a respiratory therapist I had assisted pulmonologists in bronchoscopy for many years, and could never recall doing one with a "non-pulmonologist." Not around here. So, I wasn't sure what to make of it at the time.

It just struck me as a little offbeat for a family practitioner to perform bronchoscopy, but it didn't raise any serious red flags either, and who was I to judge, anyway?

Well, not long afterward this doctor submitted an order to do a bronchoscopy on an outpatient. Furthermore, on an upcoming Saturday. Even further still, in a surgical suite. Tall orders both.

Bronchoscopy can be performed any time night or day, seven days a week, pending both routine and emergent need, but we never routinely scheduled them on a Saturday. And we absolutely never scheduled them to be performed in a surgical suite. If they were not to be performed bedside, we utilized a small low-key treatment room that was furnished for the occasion.

I called the doctor back and discussed it with him. The heretofore-atypical combination of a Saturday appointment and the reserving of a surgical suite would take some time to co-ordinate. He was insistent that it was the only day his patient was available, and that we needed to expedite the accommodations. *C'est la vie*! The surgical department thought it odd, but not totally unreasonable, though it would add an expense to the procedure, as it required the presence of an additional scrub nurse to oversee the activity in progress.

On the Saturday morning of the procedure, I had all the equipment set up in the surgical suite by eight thirty a.m. for the nine a.m. appointment. The scrub nurse was in the room with me and the doctor popped his head in at the doorway, to check on the preliminary status of everything. And immediately, he didn't just trip a couple red flags of concern, he lit off a pair of Roman candles. First, he looked over at the bronchoscope I had, that was immersed in sterilizing solution inside the Plexiglas holding tube. He said to me, "You didn't need to bring your scope. I've got my own bronchoscope in the trunk of my car. I will go down to the parking lot and get it."

What? I was immediately flabbergasted by the proposition. What physician shlubs around a bronchoscope in the trunk of his car? Does he strap it in next to the jack and the spare tire? (Houston, we have a problem.) Furthermore, he was a non-pulmonologist to boot. What was the deal here? Did this guy fancy himself some kind of swashbuckling, self-appointed, pulmonary paladin? Have scope, will travel? It was beyond odd. I had never encountered a clinical scenario like this before, but I endeavored a quick ad lib, and told him that since the procedure was being done in the hospital, we could only use hospital equipment. I didn't really know that for an absolute fact at that moment, but it sounded proper, and he immediately accepted it. Then, launching the second bizarre skyrocket, he commenced to ask the scrub nurse if she could call the laboratory and have them bring up a Bunsen burner for him to use during the procedure.

A Bunsen burner in a surgical suite?

Really? He wasn't kidding? He actually seriously requested an open-flame device to be used in the most fire-restrictive environment in the entire hospital? (Houston... Austin, Amarillo and Lukenbach, we've got a problem.)

The nurse's eyes, above her respirator mask, swelled to almost twice their normal size. She shook her head, no-no-

no, and exclaimed, "We can't use that device in here. It is totally forbidden."

I interjected and asked why would he need a Bunsen burner? He said he needed it to *heat-fix* his microscopy slides. I assured him that we always used a cold liquid fixative and that I had the requisite brushes, slides and fixative all ready to go. All fine and dandy then, he scooted off to scrub up for the procedure.

Needless to say, an unsettling feeling descended upon the room early on. Another surgical nurse soon brought in the (lightly sedated) female outpatient. She was a relatively young Hispanic lady - I think she was thirty-six - seemingly bright and healthy and sturdy. Her clinical issue was something on the order of possible throat allergy, cough, diffuse upper respiratory symptoms. Her chest X-rays were clear and no biopsies were anticipated at all. All told this had the gathering feel of an atypical, minimally justified, exploratory bronchoscopic procedure, and all of it incommensurate to the grand surgical arena.

As per protocol, with the patient settled into the surgical bed, I explained the procedure, and then began to topically anesthetize her nostrils. In this preliminary, RT-administered procedure, using a hand-bulb spritzer, an anesthetic spray is applied internally, to numb the immediate entry area inside the nose. After that, xylocaine jelly is carefully applied and advanced with long Q-tips. This serves to numb and to lubricate the nasal passage for the first few inches. Subsequently, the advancing bronchoscope will pause and deposit more numbing xylocaine (via port injections) at specific junctures moving farther down the airway. Performed with finesse, numbing and progressing, a skilled Pulmonologist can incrementally advance the scope to and through the highly sensitive vocal cords with nary a cough. Beyond the cords and larynx it is fairly clear sailing down the trachea and out into the bronchi, where much less xylocaine is required.

Unfortunately, finesse was not the coin of the realm on this occasion. The procedure began uneventfully enough. In fact, the doctor was quite conscientious in addressing any patient concerns up front. His voice was soothing and reassuring and he took extra time to make sure she was comfortable before he began. As the assistant, I had several syringes of xylocaine drawn up for the series of injections. The doctor inserted the scope properly enough, and, when the patient gagged a bit, he paused, and I reached over beside his shoulder and injected the first bolus. A little further down the patient gagged again, so another bolus was injected. (A trained Pulmonologist would better anticipate the injection locations, not necessarily wait for a gag to be the indicator. But again, gagging certainly isn't uncommon in bronchoscopy.) Eye to the scope, the doctor narrated to the patient that her nasopharynx looked good, and moving a little further in, he announced that her throat looked good, too. And then the trouble began.

Beyond the oropharynx he narrated that he could see her vocal cords. I raised up the syringe for the mandatory injection. He advanced the scope and the woman gagged and retched hoarsely. He retracted the scope a short distance and paused. I again moved the syringe up to the injection port and he tilted the scope head away, denying access. He said that she had had enough xylocaine. He didn't want her to have any more. I said, "but we need to put some on the vocal cords, especially, though." He nodded me off and then tried to advance the scope again and the woman gagged and retched like before. Then he paused again. He was apparently impatiently waiting for the previous anesthetic injections above to take hold below, which wasn't going to happen. The nurse looked at me concerned and I returned the look. I felt compelled to be more assertive. I raised the syringe up and said calmly, "we really need to put this in." This time he pushed my wrist away, looking sullen and cross. After another pause, he tried to advance the scope for a third time and the same retched gag occurred, this time getting shriller. For the fourth time I encouraged him to let me inject the xylocaine, but he was stubbornly indifferent. The scrub nurse moved around and tugged my gown and pulled me back from my position adjacent behind the doctor. The doctor continued looking in the scope but didn't advance it. She whispered tersely, "Does he know what he's doing?"

I whispered back, "It doesn't look like it. I've never worked with him before."

We rapidly agreed that, if he refused the anesthetic again, the procedure had to stop. The quick plan was for me to refuse to assist any further, and she would immediately leave and get the surgical nursing supervisor.

At the acute moment, as I returned to position behind the doctor, he was still peering into the scope intently. He no doubt had an inkling as to what our sudden sidebar entailed. He promptly withdrew the scope and then said nicely to the patient, "Unfortunately right now, your vocal cords are too swollen and edematous to continue. We will have to repeat the procedure at a later date." With that, scowling at me, he abruptly handed me the scope (thrust it into my chest) and he beat a hasty exit. The nurse and I then stood there silently flabbergasted.

Obviously, we didn't want to talk in front of the patient, so we assisted her out of the surgical suite into an adjacent recovery room bed to let her rest for a while. Back in the suite with the nursing supervisor present, we tried to reconcile what had just happened. The supervisor was incredulous when she heard about the Bunsen burner. How stupid was that? But she was obviously more concerned about the schlocky procedure that had traumatized a patient in her department. The surgery department was ultimately responsible for any maltreatment that occurred on site. Seldom performed in surgery, the nurses weren't familiar with the protocols of bronchoscopy, so it was naturally agreed that it would be my responsibility to write up a detailed incident report about the errant aspects of the procedure and the doctor's demeanor and submit it to the medical administration.

So be it. Passing no accusation or direct criticism (and not including the Bunsen burner and the bronchoscope in the car trunk—which I did relay verbally to my Pulmonary director), I wrote a methodical recap that highlighted the unsettling vocal cord sequence, and my own and the nurse's desire to halt the procedure under the circumstances. I concluded the report as the actual event *had concluded* with the doctor's truncating the procedure on his own and leaving in a brusque manner. I made one final summary suggestion that perhaps the doctor would benefit from a bronchoscopy session with one of the local pulmonologists.

Anyway, as it turned out, this new doctor had let off some adverse skyrockets in other zones as well. Independent of my submission to the medical directors, John, the pharmacy director came forward to report some highly unusual and out of bounds pharmaceutical orders from this guy. One was a bizarre (homeopathic?) concoction of Eucalyptus plants to be mushed up with other odd ball herbals that weren't part of any normal pharmacy's inventory. But the most concerning was an order for barbiturates, with a scripted dosage that was grossly, if not frighteningly over the mark. Furthermore, another nursing director on the medical floor came forward with some professional complaints of her own. All of a sudden, owing to an adverse series of unfortunate and self-inflicted events, the medical world was cratering around this doctor, and, subsequently, his temporary privileges were revoked, pending the medical board review. And, as mentioned earlier, he never showed up for it.

A short while later, my pulmonary director retroactively informed me about a few associated details of the review. Before he bolted, they did have a preliminary phone conversation with him. And he had vigorously complained that it was absolutely unacceptable for a respiratory therapist ever to sit in judgment of a doctor. (And I would eagerly concur with that sentiment. A real doctor anyway. Further, in that regard, auto-diagnostic of a real doctor is one who doesn't do anything openly derelict enough that would necessitate a therapist to sit in warranted judgement of him. But I digress.) Additionally, as the medical board had vetted him further, they later learned that he had for many years been a successful instructor at a prestigious Medical School on the East Coast. And on two prior occasions, he had tried to make the jump from academia to private practice. And, both times, the prospects had similarly failed. It appeared that moving out to the West Coast was perhaps an attempt to start anew, far away from the failures of the past. And it still didn't work. (I once heard it said, of a brainy RT whose practical skills were notably lacking, that *his intelligence ended at his elbows*. Perhaps this doctor suffered the same affliction.)

Anyway, in the instructive final analysis, from doctors to nurses to therapists, regarding any of the innumerable, hands-on procedures performed in the medical arena, competence is paramount. Staying current, staying within your practicing bounds is essential. And even then, there are times when you are off. And the wisest alternative is to defer to someone better for the moment. For example, more so in the past (before arterial lines were common place), respiratory therapists did copious arterial punctures for blood gas analysis. Poking arteries with needles is an acquired art, and some days, with some patients, for some reason, you just can't get it right. So you defer. (Luckily, for many years at Puget Sound, I was able to call in Joyce, the only RT who never misses.) Ultimately you put your ego aside, and still provide excellent care via someone else. That is the truest act of competence, and next time, it will be your turn to step in, for another highly competent compatriot who needs some help. Quality health care is always a collaborative, team effort. And ultimately, uncomfortable as it will be at the time, if something untoward and incompetent is happening to a patient, it is the clinician's obligation to step in and address it, and, if needed, stop it, report it, deal with it, fix it. Whatever it reasonably takes. As a patient care advocate, you have no choice.

You Only Live Once. The Uproarious Caper of the Boot Camp Banjo

One of the amenities of working a career in the hospital environment is that you get to meet and to know a lot of good, intelligent people, generally for a fairly long time. People interact on the job professionally, and even more so personally in the cafeteria at meal times. In my longest employment stretch as a respiratory therapist, I worked for eleven years at Puget Sound Hospital in Tacoma, WA, and over that time I grew up with the co-workers and the families with whom I worked. Coworkers' children grew from elementary kids to college kids, and experiences both happy and sad were shared. At the same time, professionally, I learned things from so many different professions beyond my own. This is where actual experience trumps educational experience in the real world. Nurses, occupational therapists, social workers, radiation specialists, surgical technicians, hospital chaplains, alcohol and drug counselors and so on, all have their own perspectives within the health care community. Without even trying, one gets a broad-spectrum glimpse into the many facets and angles of patient care that you wouldn't have ever known otherwise. And on the personal level, again, over the years, you are also treated to a lot of unique and hilarious stories that make our daily lives worth living.

I have always believed that every self-abiding, work-a-day person has at least two good novels and one good movie in their life experience. And over my thirty-year-plus career as a respiratory therapist, if I had to pick the one, most outrageously funny story that I ever heard from a co-worker, it would have to be the bodacious caper of the Boot Camp Banjo.

This uproarious true tale came from a fellow respiratory therapist named Sandy who had done a three-year hitch in the Air Force, just out of high school, way back in 1961. After joining at the recruiting center in Tacoma, he had to report to boot camp at Lackland Air Force Base in San Antonio, Texas. There was another local recruit who needed a lift to San Antonio as well, so the two of them drove all the way to Texas in Sandy's beat-up Volkswagen beetle. Little did they know what a grueling odyssey this six-week saga at boot camp would turn out to be.

Military basic training is designed to instill discipline, courage, endurance, camaraderie, and adherence to protocol. Well, as it turned out, achieving the first four of the five ideals was certainly in order. But adherence to protocol, it turns out, specifically, would a run amuck. And because of that, the first four virtues would be inculcated well beyond their imaginations.

This thick and hearty episode begins with the particular platoon of about a dozen recruits with whom Sandy found himself bunking, on the top floor of one of the two-story barracks buildings. One member of the platoon, specifically, was a Southerner whose major passion in life was playing the banjo. In fact, this good old boy considered his banjo to be an integral extension of his personality, and, like Linus' blanket, he just couldn't part with it under any circumstances. Consequently, he somehow managed to sneak his pride and joy into boot camp, and at night he would do some subdued pickin' and grinnin' for his enthralled, toe-tapping bunkmates.

One evening, however, as he was tweaking out a number, trying to keep it low, one of the bunk mates at the end near the window saw their Drill Instructor marching in through the door below. They immediately ditched the banjo and lounged back on their cots, and very soon they heard the hard, black, low-quarter shoes stomping out a number of their own up the wooden stairs. The big Sarge came to the top and barked an order, and everybody scrambled to attention at the foot of their beds. As the Sergeant passed in review between the two rows of beds and troops, he tilted his head this way and that, obviously looking for something. Upon reaching the end of the room he turned around and spoke.

I heard music up here! In fact, it sounded like a banjo playing up here! Then he demanded: *Hand it over to me right now!*

Shoulders and chins stayed tight, as eyes flashed around, and it soon became obvious that there would be no volunteers. So the determined sergeant got into the nearest recruit's face and groused,

Where's the banjo, soldier?

He responded, *No banjo, sir!*

The sergeant paused for a second and then he expanded his inquiry. He said: *It's against regulation to have any musical paraphernalia of any kind in boot camp, gentlemen. And don't tell me I'm just hearing things.*

So he barked into the next recruit's face: *Where's the record player soldier?*

No record player, sir!

Where's the radio, soldier?

No radio, sir!

We'll see about that, the sergeant assured and then he ordered every recruit to open his foot locker lid and to hold it there. The determined D.I. personally checked the interior of each footlocker visually and then physically with his foot. He ground down hard on every folded clothing item and blanket, expecting a crunch at any moment, and a big red face from the guilty party, who would then regret the error of their lying musical ways. But there wasn't a crunch in the bunch.

Frustrated, but not defeated, the sergeant assured them that they would address this issue further in the morning, and he was gone.

Early the next morning, with all the platoons and their drill instructors assembled for P.T. along the airfield, the sergeant made it a point to announce to the world that his particular group thought that boot camp was just a laid-back music session—and today, they were going to learn different. During initial P.T. Sandy's group did extra push-ups, extra sit-ups and was still running in place as the other platoons headed off for morning chow. Then, the sergeant ordered them to run two extra laps around a long tarmac area before they could go and eat breakfast—if they could get to the mess hall in time.

This punishment routine lasted for a couple of days, and then it stopped, as the issue rapidly faded. Perhaps the old Sarge figured that these young bucks had surely learned their lesson, and no doubt the radio, or whatever the musical gizmo was, had been eliminated from the premises.

Concurrently, the young troops got together to reconsider this whole musical matter carefully. For some perhaps demented reason, it was deemed kind of fun to have the irate D.I. chewing on their heads like that. You only live once, so the platoon boldly decided to advance this musical issue further, themselves. Sandy said everyone agreed to the daring caper, so they all went along with it, consequences be damned. And just for the enjoyment of their darling drill sergeant, nothing less than a robust, live performance would do.

That evening after dinner, they deliberately left the upstairs window wide open, and they waited for the D.I. to come out of the mess hall across the way. When he did, the southern boy got down and got with it and absolutely went to Nashville on the banjo—*pickin' and strummin'—wailin' and flailin'*—like Opryland on fire.

Hat scrunched in hand, the big ol' Sarge came roaring across the street like an angry, wind-milling bear. Obscenities thundered in like artillery bursts, as the livid sergeant charged, pounding his feet up the stairs. At the top, he found the men already assembled at attention, calmly looking as if nothing had happened. This was insubordination outright, and he made it a point to get real close and personal with each of them. Incensed by their daring insolence, he bellowed a lexicon that included maggots, worms and other lowly life forms, punctuated with the type of creative profanity that only real adrenaline could induce. However, despite the turbid, filthy flow of his vocabulary, the communicated demand was sparkling clear: He wanted that banjo and he wanted it—*now*.

When it again became obvious that no one would be forthcoming, the Sarge erupted, Krakatoa-volcanic. He ordered all of them to dump the entire contents of their foot lockers onto the floor; after which he personally kicked and raged and stomped through all of it, making a huge, cross-mated mess of socks, underwear, blankets and uniforms.

The footlockers were clean, so the sergeant zeroed in on what he thought for sure would be the kill. He ordered everyone to strip the pillows, blankets and sheets off of their beds and add to them to the mess; then he ordered them to lay their mattresses on the floor and to roll them up tight like a sleeping bag. No doubt one of these mattress rolls would have a large, telltale deformity to it.

G.I. bunk mattresses were not thick and cushy, by any means, and all of them rolled up into tight, uniform tubes. And the bed springs underneath were bare. The Sarge had to think some more. He stormed into the adjacent latrine and shower room and checked every nook and cranny—garbage cans, towel racks, commode lids, sink compartments, nothing. Floors and walls throughout were simple ship-lap on joists with no insulation space; there were no ceiling spaces overhead; no ventilation ducts to speak of; there was simply no place on earth to hide something as relatively big and awkward as a banjo. But it was up here somewhere. No doubt about it. And every grinning little puke knew where it was, too.

This was now war.

The physical training component got even more rigorous, and never let up. These daring young men were badgered and bullied into a physical shape none of them had known before. And over and above their intensified military training, they were molded into a potent, base-wide janitorial service as well. Not only did they routinely clean all the barracks' latrines in the evenings after dinner, the Sarge was never at a loss for creative tasks to perform during the day. Lunch times were significantly abbreviated, as the men had about two minutes to wolf down what food they could before the Sarge jerked them right back out and marched them off to perform all manners of grueling detail work. One day they might be on hands and knees in the blaring Texas sun, combing the many-acre parade field for cigarette butts, and on other days they might be in front of the base theater with chisels and putty knives, scraping melted gum wads off of the hot concrete walkways. And after that it was double-time back to the inexorable P.T. again.

This unrelenting drudgery was now their life. But it was a life of their own choosing. All they had to do to get it to stop was to turn over that banjo. Just give it up. Hand it over. They all knew where it was, and the Sarge figured at some point one of them would crack and spill the beans.

But the men kept sticking it out. And as these rough days continued for the group, they always looked forward to their one big respite. It came late in the evening, well after lights-out, when the Sarge was safely out of sight. Near drunk with exhaustion, the men would lie sprawled on their bunks, their muscles sore, their necks sunburned scarlet, and—with someone guarding the window—the southern boy would sneak the banjo out, for a soothing moment of feather-soft strumming into the night, getting ready to rest deeply and to do it all over again.

The weeks were long and miserable, but they did pass and, as the last week was nigh, the Sarge resorted to pulling surprise inspections at all hours of the night, in hopes of catching them in the act, before time ran out. On at least a few occasions, he had stood out in the dark amongst the crickets and listened to their gentle, twangy lullabies. That godforsaken banjo was up there somewhere and he just had to find it before these men shipped out. He just had to.

But it wasn't meant to be.

Basic training came to its eventual closure and the men were formally discharged from the sergeant's authority, and now had to move on to the next stages of their enlistment. A couple of these men would go off to Teletype school with Sandy, others to jet engine mechanics, still others to avionics and so forth. Accordingly, all the barracks buildings were cleared out and a series of buses had assembled to take them off to their various destinations. The several platoons of men gathered in lines with all of their carry-ons and duffel bags and so forth. And sure enough, in one of the bus lines, big as you please, the southern boy stood there, duffel bags at his side, with his sparkling-silver banjo and multi-colored strap loped across his back.

A good sport in the end, having finally spotted that infamous banjo across the distance, the Sarge moseyed over to his former group who were all milling together and making last-minute plans to keep in touch somehow. Pleasantries were exchanged and the Sarge commented that he'd had his share of clowns cycle through from time to time, but these guys were something else. He complimented them on their ability to hang tough, and figured they could probably endure a real enemy prison camp better than most. Then he looked at the banjo again and shook his head.

You guys had me half way up the nuthouse steps with this thing, he admitted, matter-of-factly.

And now that he could see the real size of the dazzling, pearl-trimmed instrument, he was even more mystified as to how they could have concealed it so well. Certainly, there had to be a logical explanation. And of course, for the sake of posterity, he felt it was only fitting for them to divulge their secret hideout.

Since the buses weren't leaving for a few more minutes, the whole jovial group—strumming banjo and all—took a stroll back down the lane and around the corner and back into the empty building that had once been their refuge, for what had seemed a whole lot longer than just six weeks.

The successful stashing of the large banjo all had to do with the stairway construction.

The open stairway that led to the upper quarters had an open wood-plank railing on the right side, and a walled-in banister on the left side with a flat hardwood cap on top. To the inside of that was a full-length, wooden handrail that was held with metal brackets. At the very top of the steps, it was demonstrated that by grabbing the top of the handrail and jerking outward, the flexible, plywood wall panel would partially release from beneath the banister cap exposing the long, narrow cavity within. With two people stationed there, it didn't take but a couple seconds to bend the sidewall open, slip the banjo inside, pop it shut and jump back into bed.

They told him, *you ran right past it every time, Sarge.*

In epilogue, as Sandy came to learn, technologically, the days of a highly-trained Teletype specialist were numbered. He did do teletype work at an airbase in Turkey for a while, but even then, the technology was changing. And after his service was completed, the transfer to a civilian Teletype career proved completely non-existent. But, in the end, that's what community colleges and respiratory therapy programs are all about. Hoo-Rah!

Hospital Workplace Violence and the Many Shades of Code Orange
A Tacoma Story

Unfortunately, a lot of things can go wrong in a hospital environment. And depending on the nature of the situation, the following examples of emergency audio alerts over the hospital intercom are fairly universal:

Code Blue (or Code 4): Cardiac-Respiratory Arrest. Send the resuscitation team.

Code Red: Fire alert in the facility

Code Gray: Suspicious person / activity at a particular location. Alerts in-house security

Code Orange: All available male help report to a particular location. It may be a fight, an unruly patient or guest, sometimes you won't know until you get there, but it is an urgency that can't be handled by routine security means.

Generally, most people would not associate hospital jobs and health care professions with a high risk of personal injury, much less risk of death. But actually (and unfortunately), hospitals and clinics are frequently places of high stress and emotion, and, not infrequently, of outbursts of violence. Families with a loved one in need of urgent care can get highly exasperated and verbally abusive if they feel that the wait is too long. And sometimes it is the nature of the patients' conditions themselves that makes them prone to unruly and sometimes violent behavior. At the very extreme, there is an ugly statistic about nurses who actually get killed on duty in hospitals by violent patients. In the vast majority of fatal assaults on RNs, the death occurs in the Emergency Department on the graveyard shift, usually by a drug-related patient. As risks for violence in the healthcare arena go, night shift in the ED is the worst of the worst, statistically. The following two citations from the same healthcare journal article elucidate this adverse healthcare phenomenon quite well.

"The average American worker stands a 1.7-in-10,000 chance of being assaulted on the job, but for registered nurses in hospitals the risk is more than tripled, at 6.1 per 10,000—higher chances of assault than faced by taxi-cab drivers or bartenders, according to the Bureau of Labor Statistics' data from 2009, the most recent available." (Carlson, J., October 17, 2011 *Critics urge execs to take safety issues more seriously;* Modern Health Care)

Needless to say, if nurses are at higher risk of assault than bartenders and taxicab drivers, something is seriously amiss. And, as summarized in the second citation, unfortunately, the dangers are almost unavoidable, due to the physical design and inherent mission of hospital facilities themselves.

"Many factors bring violence into hospitals. Jim Stankevich, the president of IAHSS, said that hospitals attract individuals who are mentally unstable, whether because of underlying psychiatric conditions, or because of the abuse of alcohol or drugs. They are open twenty-four hours, seven days a week, many times through multiple building entrances. And hospital waiting rooms are frequent sites for emotional outbursts, as overcrowding and the triage system of seeing the most acute patients first can cause long delays." (Carlson, J., October 17, 2011)

These inherent risk factors extend to all health care workers in general, but the nurses, often being the caregivers closest to the patients, naturally bear the brunt of the untoward statistics. Personally, I have witnessed numerous violent altercations in hospitals over my thirty-year-plus respiratory therapy career, especially during the eleven years for which I worked at (the now abandoned) Puget Sound Hospital in Tacoma, Washington. As outlined ahead, all of the aforementioned factors, that contribute to violence in hospitals, abounded at this facility. And when unforeseen events did get totally out of hand, the last resort was to call a *Code Orange*. (It was an urgent call for all available male help to respond to a situation in progress.)

But first, some pertinent, local Tacoma history.

As a respiratory therapist, I was hired to work at Puget Sound Hospital in the spring of 1980. Admittedly, at the time, to a certain degree, I did it for the money. It was known through the grapevine that the hospital was having serious staffing and retention problems. And, now desperate, they were acutely offering wages significantly higher than the larger medical centers in town. Money aside, it was also an intriguing opportunity to step into a struggling situation, and to try to make it a lot better. For many years back then, Puget Sound Hospital carried a lingering, dour reputation that bordered on its being the "Norman Bates

Medical Motel." It was perched on the hill at S. 36th and Pacific Avenue, overlooking the grittier center of downtown Tacoma. It was an older facility with older equipment, yet the exaggerated bad rep was truly unfair to the many fine nurses, therapists, and doctors who worked there. However, from a purely respiratory-therapy standpoint, the hospital also carried a more specific, derelict image problem.

A former RT director (a congenial guy actually), who had far too much time on his hands, couldn't resist the inane impulse to test the pH and the CO_2 level of his soda pop. So he drew up a syringe full and injected the cola sample into an expensive (thirty thousand-dollar) blood gas analyzer. Unfortunately, the intense sugar concentration of the sample gummed up the sensitive electrodes and totally fritzed the analyzer. The unit had to be taken out of service, and boxed up and sent back to the factory to be completely overhauled. As medical experiments go, this collusion of pseudo-science and soda-science was a seriously embarrassing and seriously expensive caper, to say the least. Ultimately, as a result of this poor choice by the director, the service of arterial blood gas analysis was promptly removed from the RT department, and transferred to the Hospital Laboratory. (Down the road, with our new leadership, and after some intense lobbying by our new, pulmonologist medical director, we eventually retrieved ABG analysis back to the RT department where it truly belongs.)

Anyway, this bit of *schlock-canery* with the blood gas machine became locally legendary. And well after Gary and

I had started a whole new department, we would still field some retroactive flak about it. One time, years later, I mentioned to a group of local RTs that I worked at Puget Sound Hospital and one of them responded, "Puget Sound? Oh yeah. Are you guys still doing the *Pepsi Challenge* on your blood gas machine over there?"

Like old habits, bad images die hard.

Historically, before being conjoined, the two buildings of the Puget Sound Hospital campus had remarkably different histories. The original brick building of Puget Sound Hospital was built in the early 1900s as a hospital, and the newer, adjacent concrete building was added in the early 1950s as a tuberculosis sanatorium. The two buildings were notably mismatched in style and architecture, but a fourth-floor skybridge and a ground-level breezeway were built to enjoin them. Originally the health care campus was consolidated for BN West railroad retirees. As a community medical facility, it persisted for decades as a small player in the local health care arena. But, in 1982 (much to our surprise and benefit) an ambitious, proprietary healthcare company from Dallas, Texas purchased the facility. The company immediately invested millions of dollars into extensive interior and exterior remodeling. Interestingly, they actually added cement-covered Styrofoam cornices and window frames to retro-make the newer building to look more like the older building. And for our Respiratory Therapy Department, specifically, the new owners dared us to submit a lavish wish list for everything related to our services—new modernized pulmonary lab equipment and blood gas analyzer, computerized bedside Pulmonary

Function Test equipment, updated state of the art ventilators, cardiac stress test equipment, electrocardiogram machine. The works! Wow! What a windfall! Who would have ever thought this possible when Gary and I had been hired, just two years earlier?

Gary was the director and I was the Assistant director of the department. For the first couple of years, in spite of our austere environment, we had run a very good department. We stressed super-high quality patient care, extra bedside time, and thorough family teaching. We hired only the best local RTs (Joyce in particular! Our gain was MultiCare's biggest loss.) And admittedly, we had to perform better, as a compensatory necessity to offset our less than stellar equipment. There were local doctors who were openly disgruntled at some of our antiquated pulmonary equipment. Now, at the time, Santa Claus pending, we still weren't sure if this wish list was totally for real, but we didn't hold back. We asked for the moon, and not only did the Texas folks give us the moon, they tossed in a few asteroids, to boot. All of a sudden, we were the first hospital in the region to have ventilators with a Cathode Ray (CRT) screen! This was Byzantine! We now had ventilators that outclassed those at St. Joseph's Hospital and MultiCare-Tacoma General Hospital—the two cross-town Titans of the local health care industry. (Word of caution: never be the absolute first to buy a new ventilator model—but that is another story!)

Another aspect that is worth mentioning: with the new facility upgrade came the opportunity to expand as a clinical preceptor site for the local colleges. I set up a clinical rotation for Tacoma Community College RT students, which eventually led to my getting an adjunct faculty position at the college (which I still hold all these years later). Two nurses who worked at Puget Sound likewise were teachers and preceptors for the nursing programs at Clover Park and Bates Technical Colleges. Together we freelanced some seminars and activities that really gave the students a lot of exposure and hands-on experience. As a clinical teaching facility, Puget Sound Hospital was unsurpassed. It was big enough to provide all major services, short of open heart surgery, but it was small enough that students were easily incorporated into the activity. The size and scope of our RT department was especially suited for students to get their hands on everything.

Back on topic, all told, we were feeling our new-fangled pride to be sure. Many new doctors came on board, our equipment was snazzier, and we became a noted educational site. But in the end, relative to the aforementioned risks for workplace violence and all manners of things, Code Orange, this was still Puget Sound Hospital. And that meant that we had on our fifth floor a Psychiatric Ward that contained the only involuntary lockdown facility outside of Western State Hospital. We also had a very large alcohol and drug rehabilitation unit. And, finally, we had a very active central city emergency room, just up the hill from one of the most drug-addled streets in town. All of our new and glitzy equipment was wonderful, and much of our antiquated image had been wiped away, but we were still, for lack of a better way to phrase it, *Code Orange Central*.

I couldn't begin to estimate the number of Code Orange responses I made in the eleven years I worked there, but it is easy to characterize the vast majority of them. In most cases the scenario involved a drug-rehab or psychiatric patient who was unruly and refusing to take their medications. The patient would often be seated on the floor in the hallway, refusing to return to their room. The primary objective of Code Orange is to present a passive show of force by sheer number of individuals. Respondents often numbered from six to ten, and the tactic was just casually to stand there, silent, unthreatening, not making direct eye contact with the patient, as the nurse, doctor, or mental health professional continued verbally to persuade the patient to come back to their room. Most of the time the patient benevolently relented and would join the nurse and move off, and the multi-disciplinary Code Orange respondents would naturally disperse as quickly as they had assembled.

However, sometimes the situations got far more difficult, even violent. One time, while I happened to be on location, an angry biker, wearing a spiky leather vest with dangling chains, grabbed and tried to throttle an emergency room doctor, and it quickly led to a writhing scrum pile in the ER waiting room. It took, probably, seven of us, but we eventually subdued the man and got him on a gurney with limb restraints, whereafter the police arrived and rolled him away. And in one sentinel case involving angel dust, the violent catastrophe was absolutely beyond physical belief.

Several healthcare workers were significantly injured, but no one fatally. But first, the following is a preliminary example of what constituted a highly difficult Code Orange scenario.

One time a Code Orange was called to the fifth-floor Psych Ward and six of us responded. Outside of myself, there was John, the pharmacy director (a fellow Bellarmine graduate, he '65, I '74), a couple of guys from maintenance, Jim, the central services director, and a tall red-headed guy in white bib overalls, who was the hospital painter. (Code Orange respondents are always an eclectic group.)

After being let through the big metal, double doors of the Psych Unit, the mental health professional (MHP) had us all huddle up. As the quarterback in the huddle, he warned us that this was going to be a particularly difficult task. The patient in this case was in his room, extremely agitated and defiant, verbally abusive and refusing to take his medications. His condition had been worsening throughout the day and now he was physically abusive, and a clear and present danger to the other patients and staff members. He needed to be bodily transferred from his regular patient room to a more secure lock down room. And the major complicating factor to overcome was that this violent patient was also a highly accomplished martial arts instructor. (Oh no! Combative martial arts experts off their medications? You hate it when that happens!)

As always, you follow the MHP's instructions closely. The plan was to rush into the room two rows of three abreast, and subdue him rapidly and hold him down on the bed and the MHP and his assistant would apply the four-point leather restraints. After that we would wheel him down the hallway to his new room in the adjacent lockdown section. In the assembled line up, I was in the center of the front row. John from pharmacy was to my left, and the tall red-headed painter was to my right. Correctly suspecting that the members in the first row would field some form of karate contact, the MHP had the three of us clutch bed pillows to our chests. (Turns out, what we actually needed were football helmets, but *que sera, sera*. Live and learn.)

As we gathered outside the room, already, through the small bedroom-door window, we could partially see the patient. He had moved his bed into the center of the room, and now stood atop it, shirtless, in sweat pants, in full Kung-Fu stance, knuckles folded in half, one arm extended, the other cocked back. He looked like Bruce Lee's dad, with some serious attitude. Then he came into full view as the MHP opened the door, and the three of us in the front row moved just inside the doorway restriction and briefly paused side by side. The others positioned themselves in behind us, like a wing formation. The patient stood there on the bed like a statue, stern-eyed, unflinching, not intimidated in the slightest. I kept looking at his flexed fingers; he was surely going to serve up a hard knuckle supper to someone. My exposed head began to feel like a pumpkin on a fence post at a shooting range. I inched my clutched pillow higher up on my face until it covered my nose with just my eyes peering over the top.

The MHP yelled "go!" and we surged ahead, and the patient stood frozen until the very last instant—when in a flash—he wheeled off a flying roundhouse kick. His body went airborne and his whirling heel-bone hammer came around like a comet. God knows that the driving heel point would have seriously imploded the right side of my head if it hadn't been for the painter's head being perfectly in the way. "Swack!" The painter went down in a heap, and the recoil of the leg off of the painter's head caused the airborne patient to fall sideways down on to the mattress. I leaped on to his midsection with my pillow and John leaped on to his upper body and suddenly the others had his four limbs held, and the MHP dutifully applied the four-point restraints pronto. Done. The entire, active, takedown process took maybe thirty seconds at most. It actually went like clockwork, except for the unfortunate painter, who was now in a different time zone.

With the patient safely secured for the moment, all attention shifted to the crumpled painter on the floor. He was groggy and weak, but able to sit up and to get his bearings. He was officially done painting for the day. We got a wheelchair and took him down to the emergency room, where he spent the rest of the shift napping on a gurney while being observed for signs and symptoms of concussion. All told, he didn't just take one for the team, but he took one for me personally. Had he managed to duck in time, I would have been the one convalescing in the emergency room. Purple Hearts are not awarded for Code Oranges, but the painter certainly deserved one.

Circa 1990, the worst Code Orange of all time for me involved an angel dust incident that, to this day, still boggles my mind. I still can't reconcile the physical manifestation of the event. Most everyone has heard some tale about the super-human strength that angel dust victims can generate. This is a gigantic case in point. There was no video camera in the facility to record the specifics of the event, and all that the few, bruised and battered witnesses could say about it was that, "he simply did it."

This uproarious incident happened on a sedate Sunday evening, but some related details of the story had actually begun on the Friday evening before. I was working the swing shift on the previous Friday, and was also scheduled to work the upcoming weekend. I got a routine call to perform an electrocardiogram on the fifth floor. Again, the fifth floor was a "psychology ward" but it was divided between the "serious lock-down section" and the more routine "counseling section," if you will. And this electrocardiogram patient will serve to typify the difference.

As one exited the elevator on the fifth floor, immediately to the right stood the imposing, double metal doors of the psych unit. Each door had a very small wire-reinforced window to view through. There was a huge stainless steel electronic bolt latch, that locked the doors in the middle, and to the right side was a built-in speaker system that allowed you to identify yourself and to communicate with the nursing station, just inside, across the hallway. On that Friday evening, I was allowed entry with my EKG machine. I took a left turn, and went down the hallway to the "routine section." At the room in question, I found a solitary, shirtless, African-American male sitting up in bed. I confirmed his name, explained the process and proceeded to attach the EKG sensor wires to his arms and legs. Concurrently, it was impossible for me not to comment on the man's physique. His ripped body was an artwork of chiseled black marble; his spectacular muscle definition bespoke many hours in the gym. I said in passing admiration, "obviously you are a body builder; you must work out quite a lot."

He responded somewhat downheartedly. "Well yeah, I work out a lot. Actually, I am a professional football player. A full back. I've never been cut from a team in my life, but last week I was the very last one cut from the final roster of the Seahawks."

He then went on to confide that he had a new fiancée, and her young kids, and that they were planning a whole new life together. The woman and her children had relocated to the area to carry on with his professional career, and the team cut had totally thrown his life into chaos. The fiancée was forced to move back in with her parents, in another state, while he tried to secure his future options in football. He was hopeful that it would all work out in the long run, but right now he was really down and having a tough go of it, so the team doctor suggested that he get some rest and recreation in the meantime. And so here he was, temporarily battling a major life setback, but determined to get back to the NFL in short order. He wanted to get his new family back together as soon as possible. And to that end I wished him god's speed.

After the EKG, we chatted some more about football and weightlifting routines and so forth, and then I eventually headed out.

About forty-eight hours later, it was a rainy Sunday evening, about five thirty p.m. Swing shifts on Sundays in a hospital are often desolate affairs. The hospital is void of nearly all department supervisors and administrators, with only a skeleton crew of maintenance workers and receptionists. I was walking by myself through the ground level breezeway when the Code Orange was called. And it was not a typical, terse, methodical announcement. It was a desperate shrieking announcement—a female voice pleading "Code Orange - fifth floor - please help! Please! Fifth floor..." There was some frantic scuffling, and the announcement was cut off.

Whoah! This was definitely not good!

Chilled, I ran to the first-floor elevator, just sixty feet ahead of where I was walking. I punched the up button and waited. I looked both ways up and down the hallway: not a soul to be seen. Obviously, something traumatic was occurring upstairs, and I hoped there would be additional respondents. It seemed that I was the only person on the main floor of the hospital. The elevator arrived, and I jumped in and punched #5, the top floor. When the doors parted, I began to step out quickly—teetering forward—but caught myself and stepped back, nearly losing my balance. The sight was inexplicable. Lying flat on the hard marble-like floor in front of the elevator were the two giant metal doors of the Psych unit. The metal doors had been ripped from the surrounding metal frame. I could immediately see the out-puckered screw holes in the metal frame, where the large machine screws once had secured the hidden hinges in place. On the floor, some of the bent hinges still had the big, also-bent screws poking out of them: metal screws ripped from metal threads on both massive doors at once. (Had a rhinoceros crashed through here?)

The only way to move ahead was to walk on and over the doors themselves, so I did. At the open frame entrance, I began to take a right turn, and again had to stumble to a stop. Just around the corner to the right, the charge nurse Brenda was seated on the floor, her back upright against the wall. She looked up at me forlorn, her face bruised and I could see blood trickling out of the right corner of her mouth. I dropped down to a knee and asked if she was all right. It was obvious she was dazed, voice breathless, but she waved me off assuredly, "I'll be OK, I'll be OK." Then she lifted her arm and pointed her finger to an entrance way across the hall. It was the entrance way that led to the small patient cafeteria. "He's in there. He's in there," she repeated, then she put her arm down.

Still kneeling, I looked over. He's in there. My mind searched in a flash—who was he in there? And what was going on here? And who, in god's name, had been strong enough to rip down metal doors like this? I stood up and began to head for the hallway, and then the memory struck me. The Seahawk guy! An NFL fullback. He was about as strong and physically imposing a person as I had seen in a long while. Maybe he had gone berserk? Maybe he had just shoulder-plowed through those doors like he was blasting through a wall of linebackers? My heart pounded with fear, as I headed down the short hallway. Already I could hear a groaning, struggling altercation in progress. And when I took the left turn into the enclosed cafeteria, the scene was right out of a movie. Some patients were up on the countertops while others were kneeling on table tops; all were trying to avoid the violent fracas taking place on the floor.

As it turned out, the powerful Seahawk guy was thoroughly involved in the situation, but not to the extent hypothesized. Lying sideways on the floor, the Herculean Seahawk clung to a small, 145-pound, bearded, wild-eyed man, holding him in a desperate leg lock and arm lock at the same time. Grunting in a shrill, savage manner, the bearded man's trapped body surged and flexed and lurched, each time dragging the clinging Seahawk another foot or two across the floor. I nervously circled the imbroglio from above, not knowing what at all to do. The Seahawk grimaced at me and squeaked, almost in tears, "I can't hold him much longer." I literally turned circles, not knowing what to. I couldn't bash the guy in the head and try to knock him out; I didn't have any rope to tie him up; I didn't perceive any way for me to get down on the floor and to help hold him in place. The whole thing was crazy wacko awkward.

Thankfully, at that moment the MHP rushed in, syringe in hand. He was the main MHP with whom I had worked for many years. He was a strong, stocky baldheaded man, who walked with a distinct limp. And today his bald white head was splotched with deep red and purple bruises. Obviously, along with Brenda, he had taken some punishing blows. Immediately he knelt down, grabbed some arm flesh and injected the tranquilizer pronto. (And no, he didn't pause to use an alcohol prep pad; sometimes standard protocol can wait.)

The injection acted quickly, and the writhing struggle stopped. The Seahawk was finally able to release and he rolled to the side and on to his back, where he lay panting for a while, trying to catch his breath. Additional help and a security guard arrived, and they assisted the MHP in relocating the sedated patient to a lockdown room. Shortly, I extended an arm, and helped bring the Seahawk upright off the floor, after which he had a seat in the nearest chair. It was now safe for the frightened patients to come down off the countertops and tabletops. They offered some kudos to the exhausted Seahawk, some applauded and others patted him on the back as they headed out.

Still puzzled by it all, the Seahawk looked at me and said, incredulously, "You know, I have been in some head-to-head fights with NFL linemen before. And I've scrapped it up with some bad boy linebackers, too. But I'll tell you what, that little guy was the baddest dude I've ever tangled with in my life. Wow, he was strong! He must have been on something!"

Turns out he was on something. Angel dust.

I hung around the unit in the aftermath a while longer, actually hoping to assuage my curiosity about the demolished doors again. What had he done? Had he taken a running body slam into them? Or had he squatted down and bench pressed the door handles, like some kind of human demolition jack? I stood there looking perplexed at the flattened doors, and one of the male nurses came walking by, and I asked, "how did he actually do this?"

A bit distracted, and not much in the mood to talk about it right then, he said, "he just did it, man. He just did it." And he walked on.

Shortly thereafter, I walked on too, ever curious about what physical sequence had actually taken place in the tearing down of those heavy steel doors.

In the final analysis, taking all personal experiences to a larger, general level, nursing and allied healthcare professions make for great careers, and I would eagerly recommend them to any young people starting out, or to older, experienced people looking to go back to school for a new career. And a key word and active goal in all modern patient care is collaboration. It embodies teamwork among the many disciplines to combine their efforts for the sake of better patient outcomes. It means being on your toes and looking for anything advantageous to the patient and their families. The satisfaction of working with people and families can be heartfelt. Unfortunately, on a few untoward occasions, it means teaming up to deal with something unexpectedly difficult, and maybe even violent. Risks of violence in the workplace go with just about any industry, healthcare especially included. Healthcare facilities have some added degrees of difficulty that require a rapid response and careful teamwork that serves everyone well in a pinch. Code Orange. There are many shades to it. And you hate to hear it. But your healthcare comrades depend upon your responding to it.

A Demonic Encounter: A Patient Deeply Possessed of Mind and Numerous Bullet Fragments

When it comes to occupations in which workers can say "they've seen it all," for several reasons, few occupations can compete with respiratory care. From home care to hospital care, from adult care to neo-natal care, respiratory therapists are actively engaged in clinical service all across the modern healthcare arena. From the emergency room to the critical care unit, from the patient care floors to the outpatient clinics, from the pulmonary exercise labs to the overnight sleep labs, RTs directly interact with numerous patients at many different clinical levels and disease states. And demographically, as grim distributors of people in need of care, the twin scourges of disease and misfortune cut about as wide a swath across humanity as anything. And, in deference to Mr. Murphy (what can go wrong will) people themselves can be highly susceptible to odd and untoward health care events.

Consequently, all that considered, given their broad spectrum of patient exposure, from hospitals to homes, it is especially common for RTs to observe a large share of unusual patient-care predicaments and follies. Ultimately, there is no telling what an average RT will experience on a given work shift, especially at night with a full moon overhead! The following case is a good example.

This disastrous, convoluted patient-care episode took a while accurately to reconstruct. Luckily there were no fatalities. Although pharmaceutical in its inception, strangely enough, it invokes a real-world parallel to the paranormal topic of demonic possession. Of all the potential pathological human maladies to be had in our ocean of air (rational and irrational), the prospect of demonic possession is probably the most hideous of all to contemplate. Even if you don't believe in it, it still scares the heck out of you to read about it or to watch it on the movie screen. Sensationalized long ago by the movie THE EXORCIST, the alleged gory symptoms of satanic takeover—i.e., rotating heads, outbursts of profanity, projectile barfing and what not—have become stereotypical to most people. However, this issue and its many ramifications are far older than Hollywood, and in some countries clashes have occurred between the church and the government on how best to deal with the supposedly possessed victims. In Germany, for example, Christian authorities are not allowed to perform exorcisms on people without medical intervention first, to rule out and to treat possible organic syndromes—severe epilepsy, in particular. I've read that there are documented cases of severe epilepsy in which many of these associated horrendous symptoms have occurred. These symptoms include fiendish voice and behavior changes, bizarre vomiting episodes, and even gory musculo-skeletal contractions so severe that actual arm, leg and finger joints are repeatedly dislocated and relocated—snapping and popping— as the rhythmic muscles contort wildly out of control.

A somatic event as graphic as this would be deeply unsettling to witness, even for experienced medical personnel. But the one consolation of sorts is that the victims of such organic anomalies typically have no memory of the acute, spastic episodes. And that is the critical element that prevails in this episode—*memory*, which is functionally synonymous with awareness and self-control. Whether the devil be real or clinically metaphorical, the prospect of having one's mind and body possessed by an alternate force that violently directs your actions without your being aware of it has to be one of the most frightening aberrations to consider in the inventory of human experience. In the following real episode of such an event, the only devil is in the details, but, as usual, real-world clinical events provide real-world lessons for all concerned.

Circa 1986, this violent conundrum begins around midnight as an angry man in his mid-twenties is brandishing a loaded pistol and screaming and kicking against a downstairs apartment door, threatening to shoot and kill all the people inside. He had warned them earlier that he would come back to get them, and, quite obviously, he meant it. Meanwhile, on the other side of the battered door, the once-jovial party folks now scrambled desperately to stack chairs and couches against the door, to keep the enraged gunman from entering. The police had already been called.

Suddenly, in the parking lot directly behind the fanatical gunman, a police patrol car roared in and skidded to a stop. The patrol car doors flew open, and, with weapons drawn, the two officers ordered the man to drop his gun and to lie down. In a jolt of rage, without aiming, the gunman swung the pistol toward the policemen and fired a shot and then he turned and ran. As the wild shot struck one of the tires on the police car, one of the officers returned a single shot that hit the fleeing gunman in the right shoulder blade region and dropped him. Immediately thereafter, the officers converged, confiscated the weapon and promptly radioed for an ambulance.

The ambulance responded quickly, and rushed the gunman to a nearby hospital where he was surgically treated for severe chest wounds. He had sustained multiple lung punctures and other internal damage, including sundry fragments of bullet casing that were lodged too closely to his spine and other organs to bother extracting. All in all, though, the surgery went so well that the damaged lungs re-inflated nicely, with chest tubes in place, and (somewhat amazingly) the still-anesthetized man breathed well enough on his own that he did not require a mechanical ventilator. His immediate prognosis was much better than expected, under the circumstances, and, of course, the police had to wait until the anesthesia wore off before they could question the man and get some broader detail on the whole miserable situation.

At the same time, the wounded man's incredulous parents arrived at the hospital and were equally interested in questioning their son. This was absolutely unbelievable to them. This just could not happen to their boy. He had been too good, too nice, too free of trouble his whole life. How in the land of Goshen could their son perpetrate the diabolical acts of threatening to kill an apartment full of people, and then get into a shootout with the police? And now they see him in a hospital bed, surrounded by police guards, with all four of his limbs chained to the bed frame! Preposterous! Of course all parents want to give their children the benefit of the doubt, but in their minds, this nightmare was impossible. It was categorically beyond the *Outer Limits* for this to be happening. They anxiously waited for their son to wake up and to explain his catastrophic actions...

Meanwhile, to segue back and then ahead in time, there was a fine young man in his mid-twenties who had developed an internal abdominal disorder that was treatable with special medication. However, it was imperative that this medication *not be mixed with alcohol*, lest any number of untoward physiological reactions manifest.

Well, this nice person was invited to a party, so he went, and while he was there he figured (unwisely) that one drink couldn't hurt. So he had one. And it wasn't long before this person became agitated, and then downright obnoxious to the other party guests. He wasn't behaving at all like the bosom buddy everyone knew. But because they all liked him, they cut him some slack and gave him another drink, to help him chill out; and then he became so grossly, verbally offensive to everyone that they had no choice but to ask him to leave. This only served to enrage him further still, so finally, everyone just bodily ushered him out the door. Wolf-eyed with fury, he made it patently clear that he was going home to get a gun and would return to get them all...

Perspectives being different for different observers, a fine young man went to a friend's party one night, and, after his first drink, his only memory was that of dozing off into a deep slumber. Then he awoke the next morning to find himself in foreign environs, body heavily bandaged, suction tubes snaking out of his chest, with all four of his limbs cuffed and chained to the bed. A chilling disorientation, but he quickly realizes that somehow, some way, he has ended up seriously injured in a hospital bed. And of all the interested parties hovering over him—he is the most stymied of all—and begins pleading for someone to tell him what had happened.

He took the words right out of their mouths. They were hoping he could tell them. Yet, after a series of questions by the police, it became readily apparent that he really had no clue at all as to what had transpired. He vaguely remembered the party; he had no memory of leaving, no memory of shooting the gun, no memory of having been shot himself. Eventually, after some additional sequential reconstruction, it didn't take too long to figure out the drug-reaction conundrum. At that point, the police realized they weren't dealing with a *real criminal threat* here, so they removed the four-point restraints, and the whole atmosphere surrounding the situation relaxed.

Circumstantially, this wasn't really premeditated, attempted murder, nor was it really shooting at a police officer, so to speak. It was a freak drug reaction that had happened to a thoroughly scrupulous person who was oh-so-lucky to be alive. The parents were ever so thankful, all the way around, and by and by, as all the pieces fell into place, the police assured them that nothing seriously punitive would likely become of this unfortunate incident. But, at the moment, for legal purposes, until the official paperwork finally cleared, the police still had to keep their son under perfunctory guard, which meant that an officer had to be stationed at the location round the clock.

And of course, this wasn't such a bad assignment for the cops in question, as they got to lounge around the hospital room with the wounded guy and to read the newspaper and to watch TV and so forth. (It was no doubt a welcomed change from those many other occasions where real violent offenders are held under hospital guard—two-hundred-and-fifty-pound Charles Manson types—who need to have someone watch them like a hawk, in spite of the four-point restraints.)

In fact, as a humorous aside, given the laid-back situation in the room, this story took an awkward twist one morning, as a respiratory therapist had walked in while the police guard and the wounded guy had been deep into a discussion about salmon fishing. The policeman himself had proudly bragged that, just a few mornings ago, he had caught four big silvers off of the north side of Fox Island. When the respiratory therapist casually pointed out that the daily limit was *two* salmon, the cop recovered smoothly by pointing out that he had made two trips, one before sunrise, one after. From a "solaristic" standpoint it might as well have been separate days...

Yeah, right.

Anyway, the real world was certainly back to normal, it would seem, and that would basically conclude the clinical elements of this very real and death-defying type of *pharmaco-demonic possession*. The immediate pharmaceutical takeaway is never to mix alcohol with drugs that expressly warn you not to do so on the label! Just don't do it! And for clinicians, when formulating care plans and teaching patients about proper drug use at home, it is imperative that both the patient and the family are appraised of the potential dangers.

But—truth being stranger than fiction again—there was an interesting and off-the-wall social and technical sequel to this shooting event, as well.

A few days later, very early in the morning, a well-dressed official came into the hospital, and first met with the surgeon who had performed the lifesaving operation. The two of them meticulously preened over the X-rays of the patient's body before and after the surgery, and then they catalogued all manners of the external and internal wounds. After that, they went into the room and had the wounded man sit up, where they then proceeded to peel back the bandaging in order to inspect the wounds visually.

It was at least marginally impolite for the inspecting official not to introduce himself, and at some point the wounded man casually inquired if he was a new doctor on the case.

The official replied that, *no, he was not a doctor.* And then he didn't follow up, apparently hoping to leave it at that.

The inspection continued and the wounded man's curiosity grew so he then asked the official *what was it that he did do?*

Again the response was brief and dangling: *I uh, I work for the police department.*

Another long pause commenced, and since that was all that was forthcoming, the next logical question of course was, *what do you do for the police department?*

Realizing that he could not properly maintain a professional anonymity under these circumstances, the official reluctantly relented... *well, I was hoping not to go into it, but... if you really want to know... I am a ballistics expert. And... .um... recently, I got the local police department to switch over to a new kind of bullet. And uh... as it turns out... you are the first person that we shot with it. And, I now have to do a follow up to see how well our new bullet worked.*

Now, most people may not have been all that interested in the specific technical properties of a police bullet that had nearly claimed their life, but the wounded man found the topic acutely fascinating and wanted to know all about this *new kind of bullet.*

And now that the ice had been broken and the ballistics expert did not need to be self-conscious about his craft, he was delighted to delve into the minutiae of his trade, and a really chipper discussion soon followed. Adding some levity, the parenthetical jibes are my own, but the serious gist of the discussion could be condensed as follows.

One of the problems confronting the police, whenever they returned gunfire in urban settings, was that the old, standard, solid-lead slugs were prone to going through the bad guys (*who are innocent until proven guilty, but only after they've stopped shooting, and if they're still alive*) and striking innocent bystanders, on the periphery of the crime scene. What was needed was a less-solid, lighter-weight, more disintegrating type of bullet that would enter a body but not go all the way through it, thus reducing peripheral bystander risk (*and economically containing all invested energies within the criminal portfolio*). So now enters this newly developed police ammunition (*much more urbane, lighter, faster, perhaps the Perrier of contemporary bulletry*), which has a deep, hollow-point configuration, with a special type of rapid-expanding jacket. The bullet structure was designed to penetrate the body, split asunder at the seams, scatter apart into pieces and remain there inside the body. And all told in that regard, since there were indeed several bullet fragments still lodged inside the wounded man's body, and since there was no exit wound in front, all indications were that this nouveau-ammo *really really worked!*

High fives weren't quite in order (especially with chest tubes in place), but the ballistics expert was gratified with the results, and the wounded man, a good sport to be sure, was impressed as well. (*Few people, I suppose, are ever so intimately and physically acquainted with their own tax dollars at work.*)

In the final analysis, the long-standing axiom prevails, that truth is far stranger than fiction. And, given all the possible tragic outcomes contained within this violent episode, from the scene at the apartment, to the shot at the police, to the severe wounds inflicted by the return fire, to the timely transport to surgery and so forth, in spite of the ersatz state of demonic possession, the devil had no hand in on this one. In fact, everyone involved in this potentially catastrophic event was able to relish a happy ending. The threatened party-goers were unharmed. The wounded son survived. The parents' desperate hopes were vindicated as to the son's innocence and untarnished reputation. The police actions were entirely commendable, as they responded quickly, they didn't fire until fired upon, and then they were swift in getting the wounded assailant to the hospital. In fact, it was an impeccable job by law enforcement all the way around. And finally, in the ceremonious end, like a proud papa, the ballistics expert could now pass out cigars to celebrate the baptism of his new bullet baby!

Love You to Death. Until We Do Part

This thought-provoking story is unsettling to recount. It is a little bit Hitchcock, a little bit Twilight Zone. Ironically, it is a thoroughly uplifting and inspiring account of a loving and caring couple. Yet, in resolution, it is a heartrending enigma as well. This whole healthcare episode has a ponderable perplexity about it that lingers awkwardly in the mind.

This story came to me from a fellow respiratory therapist named Sandy (the same Sandy of the Boot Camp Banjo imbroglio in another story). Earlier in his career he, too, had worked for a respiratory homecare company, and had covered a lot of territory in his rounds. Well before the era of CPAP machines, his home patient mix included oxygen services, small- volume nebulizers, IPPB machines and tracheostomy care. He single-handedly covered the whole southwest sector of Washington state, from I-5 west to the ocean. And this patient care story revolves around a husband and wife who lived way out in a remote area on the Washington coast. The wife was the afflicted one, suffering from severe COPD, and utilizing twenty-four-hour oxygen service and nebulized bronchodilator treatments. Sandy's monthly visit to this location was one of the longest drives he had to make from Tacoma, but he said that the trip was always worth it. This couple was the quintessential storybook pair who carried their romance well into the golden years, despite any disheartening medical condition. Always smiling and thankful, the slender wife was frail in appearance but still ambulatory, yet the husband insisted on using a wheelchair to port her around most of the day. Inside the small, ornate, Bavarian-style home, the fifty-foot nasal tubing line on the oxygen concentrator allowed her to reach most of the locations in the house. And, for outdoor travel, the wheelchair had sleeved pockets on the back, into which the portable oxygen tanks could fit. Accoutered as such, they traveled locally, they attended movies, they took strolls on the idyllic beach just beyond the home. Except for the miniscule distraction and inconvenience of the medical equipment, they lived life as they would have otherwise. And the driving force behind that was the husband's relentless ingenuity and driven Germanic determination.

A real-life Disney Geppetto with thick white hair and mustache, the husband was a sturdy, ever-jolly, soft-spoken craftsman of Bavarian descent. His talents were numerous, woodworking, particularly. He had built their chalet-style home himself, and the surrounding lawns and gardens were adorned with his handmade windmills, birdhouses and trellises of grape vines and climbing roses. Day-to-day, with his wife's needs thoroughly attended-to for the moment, he prodigiously indulged his passions of woodworking, pastry baking and sausage making. Sandy recalled that he couldn't leave after his monthly visits without accepting a generous load of spicy German sausages, along with a box of the pastry de jour. One month the pastry might be baklava, another month raisin bread, and his favorite pastries were the sticky, gooey, frosted German cinnamon rolls called *Schnecken*. (The German word for *snail*.) Disastrously hyper-calorific, some of the heavily glazed cinnamon rolls were plain, some were crusted with pecans, and Sandy assured me that these coiled, puffy, glistening treats had no equal on this planet. And of course, Sandy was not the only recipient of this culinary largesse, because no visit to the pulmonary clinic would be complete without a large complement of the same goodies for the doctors, nurses and clinic workers. He was legendary in his own right, and of course, everywhere they went, the wife was wont to point out how lucky she was to have such a man caring for her. A gift from heaven he truly was.

    A great deal of this man's ability to tend to so much business at once—I guess we would call it multi-tasking today—was his penchant for ingenuity and efficiency. His wife's medical care plan involved taking many medications at specific time intervals, so he constructed a long-legged, wooden pharmaceutical cabinet, with glass doors to hold all the medications in full view and within easy reach from a wheelchair. The cabinet had shelves, to hold all the medicine containers label-out, and the tilted bottom shelf had seven little box sections, to hold each day's set of pills, complete with a note on the times to take the inhaler medications stationed on the shelf directly above. The little notes were discarded after each use, so that there was no ambiguity about the medication's having been forgotten or not. Forgetting to take medications, or accidentally doubling up on medications, is a common, long-standing problem with elderly patients. But not in this household.

The husband meticulously oversaw the filling of the boxes each week, and the detailed care plan schedule was ticked off each day with a watchmaker's zeal.

All in all, Sandy couldn't help but be enamored of this wonderful couple, and who couldn't be thoroughly impressed and amazed by the husband's pervasive love and care? Most important, in Sandy's view, was the ever-positive nature of the emotional support. On his visits, they always took some leisure time to converse on the living room sofa, or at the dining table with snacks, or all three might go for a short walk in the garden, weather permitting. And always the mood was happy and upbeat. On one visiting occasion, however, table-side, while seated in her wheelchair, the wife appeared a little shorter of breath than usual. She took to performing her pursed lip breathing maneuver. It is a tactic which aids in oxygenation by back pressuring the lungs and keeping the smaller airways open. It is an overt breathing maneuver, and it interferes with conversation a little bit; and the wife self-consciously sighed and then she openly lamented the years during which she had smoked cigarettes. If only she hadn't smoked. She wouldn't be a burden to anyone. Always ameliorative, the husband calmly diverted her from her downward mood, and assured her that there was no reason to be regretful of the past. After all, both had been smokers; either one of them could have been victimized by it. And, most importantly, he insisted, by no means was she a burden. Years ago, when the wife had been diagnosed with COPD, both had quit smoking together. Quitting smoking is always a good choice, and often there is a notable improvement in health afterwards; but sometimes the damage done is not forgiving. But not to worry, from the husband's perspective. All that mattered was that they were together.

Immediately, the wife's spirits brightened up and she smiled again. In her soft voice, she indirectly praised, and thanked her husband by asking Sandy if he had ever seen or known such a wonderful man? After swallowing his gooey, heavenly mouthful of *Schnecken*, Sandy sincerely admitted that he had not.

In the end, we are all human and we are all mortal, and this reality is probably impressed upon home healthcare workers more than anyone else. For homecare RTs, the notification that someone you knew and cared for has passed on usually comes in a blunt, non-descript invoice to pick up the respiratory equipment at a suddenly-recognized name and address. The one and only reason to pick up oxygen equipment is because it is no longer needed. Good news for some. But for elderly, end-stage (incurable) COPD patients, the reason that the life-sustaining equipment is no longer needed is a heartbreak that speaks for itself.

When Sandy got the order to pick up the woman's oxygen equipment out on the coast, he was mortified. For the moment, he didn't know what to do. He thought about calling the husband ahead of time, but he didn't have a clue what to say at the moment. At least the long drive out there would give him time to contemplate his words, and hopefully he could be as consoling to the husband as he had always been to the wife. He couldn't help but think how lonely it would be for him now, way out on the remote beach road. For the last several years, all his activities had circulated around his wife and her medical needs and doctors' appointments. Even most of his creative baking and sausage making was done for the benefit of others involved in her care. All things considered, he figured the husband, a proud German man, might be outwardly stoic, but, inside, he would be devastated. Still uncertain of what to say and how to say it, he decided just to let the words flow when he talked to him. He dutifully headed out of Tacoma, southbound on I-5.

Two hours later he pulled into the driveway.

Heart in his throat, Sandy knocked on the door. The door soon opened and to Sandy's surprise greeting him there was a well-dressed woman. A relative perhaps? Then he realized it was the wife. Lip stick on, her hair done up nicely, he barely recognized her. She looked chipper and spry in her floral dress, with no wheelchair in sight. She thanked him for coming and led him inside, indicating that the equipment was just down the hallway in the utility room. Stupefied, Sandy followed her as she scooted ahead, with her heeled shoes cluck-clucking on the hardwood floor. At the utility room entrance they paused, and Sandy could see the equipment—the concentrator and oxygen tanks neatly stacked together, ready to go. At a struggling loss for words now, he first mumbled incoherently, then swallowed, and asked, self-consciously, "uhm, so you don't need the oxygen anymore?"

She responded, "Since the tragedy, I found out that I really didn't need it."

"Tragedy?"

She recounted, "Oh, I am sorry. I thought they told you. My husband suddenly passed away with a heart attack, about a month ago."

Breathless, Sandy sought to console her but she patted his arm and assured him that all was OK, and she was getting along well despite the tragic loss. She reiterated that her husband was the most wonderful man in the world, and that when he had passed, she completely panicked and didn't know what to do. Family and friends immediately filled in, but, given the inevitable, she simply had to learn to do more things for herself now, regardless of her medical condition. And the more she *did do* for herself, the more she quickly learned what she *could do* for herself. The more she walked around on her own, the more she realized that she didn't need the wheelchair. She took some long walks on the beach without the oxygen, and got a little short of breath, but not disastrously so. She didn't know what her physical limits were, but she had never tried testing her physical limits, either. Years ago, the doctors had said that her lung condition was terminal, and they had completely accepted it. And they had fully accepted the life-changing roles that came with it. Her husband relished his role as the caretaker, and so did she. He so thoroughly took care of everything that she didn't have to think about it. And that was all fine and well, because, as far as she knew, she *truly was* sick. But then he died, and she suddenly had to take care of herself; and she found, to her great surprise, that maybe she wasn't nearly as helpless, nor as terminal, as she had thought. (Or had been taught to think by the doctor? Or was she playing a role that pleased her husband?) She didn't have an explanation for it. But in just a few weeks, the more she walked, the easier it became, so she just quit using the oxygen altogether. She had finally got tested again a few days previously, at the doctor's office, and she did well enough that the doctor submitted the order to discontinue the oxygen service. Additionally, she was going to further explore how many of the medications she could discontinue as well. Maybe she didn't need those either.

Sandy was still trying to process it all in his head, when she looked at her watch, and announced that she was running late. She hated to shoo him out, but she had a plane to catch in a few hours, and needed to meet up with her girlfriends. She concluded the conversation by saying somberly, "I'll miss my wonderful husband forever. But life does go on." Then she spanked her hands together and zoomed a palm upward and chirped, "Right now I'm catching up on some lost time. Me and the girls are *flyin' to Reno*!"

Sandy quickly gathered up his emotions along with the respiratory equipment, packed it all into his vehicle, and had a long introspective drive home.

The Nexus of Wolff-Parkinson-White Syndrome and a Discounted Refrigerator Repair Job

You just never know when a little bit of medical knowledge can come in handy and greatly benefit you in a time of need. Granted, there is a very large gap between congenital myocardial conduction defects and a major refrigerator repair job, but I was able to capitalize on that very juncture. Here is the story in full.

First, as a respiratory therapist who worked for several hospitals wherein the RT department was responsible for performing EKG tracings, I took it upon myself to be an aficionado of electrocardiography, including learning some detailed history on the pioneers of our current knowledge of various cardiac dysrhythmias and syndromes. Pertinent to the story here is that, in the 1920's, doctors Wolff and White (both researchers from Boston University) were studying a peculiar cardiac phenomenon. As related ahead, there were people who had an extra little bump in their EKG wave form. This little bump occurred between the p-wave (atrial activation) and the QRS wave (ventricular activation.) Normally there is a distinct, flat pause between these wave forms, denoting no electrical muscle activity at all. But something was triggering the heart muscle early; there was a small quiver of muscle activity *when and where* there wasn't supposed to be any; but there were no symptoms to this specific configuration. By itself, the wave form was benign. The heart pumped blood just fine. But it became known that many people who had the little bump wave were predisposed to wild bouts of sudden tachycardia—the heart racing out of control—oftentimes exceeding two hundred and fifty beats per minute. During these bouts, the EKG rhythm was a frantic up and down wave form that perfectly mimicked a dangerous, life-threatening rhythm called ventricular tachycardia (V-tach). These "bump-wave" tachycardia events were frightening and unnerving for the victims, but they weren't at all as life-threatening as real V-tach. Eventually, the tachycardia episode would subside, and the patient's wild rhythm would shift back (convert) to their normal EKG rhythm, with the added little bump in it.

What was the deal with the bump wave here? How did it contribute to the heart's shifting in and out of tumultuous tachycardia like that? Wolff and White wanted to know. They set up a laboratory, and got numerous patients (who had the little bump wave—now called a Delta wave) to volunteer hours of time on EKG machines, racking up miles of EKG strip paper, in hopes of catching the tachycardia transition in the act. Of course, there were no electronic, telemetric monitors back then, which would have made the research a whole lot easier. But coincidentally at the time, in the medical literature they came across the writings of a Dr. Parkinson; he was a medical researcher from London who turned out to be studying the very same cardiac conundrum. Ultimately, they got into contact with each other, via mail, and they decided to form a *trans-Atlantic* alliance. The American researchers and the English researchers would share all their study information, tactics and findings, and would, hopefully, expedite a resolution to this mysterious, fluctuating, cardiac syndrome, henceforth called Wolff-Parkinson-White Syndrome, or WPW for short.

To summarize the anatomical cause, about one in three hundred hearts is born with a tiny, residual strand (or strands) of cardiac muscle fiber that connects the top portion of the heart (atrial muscle and chambers) to the larger bottom portion (ventricular muscle and chambers), and acts as an accessory pathway for muscle stimulation. The little muscle strip connections are left-over fragments from way back in the gestation period—about eight to ten weeks post-conception. Back then, the four developing muscle chambers of the heart are all interconnected, wobbling around with little coordination, and a cartilage structure quickly forms between them. The cartilage mass grows outward from the middle, forming the four cardiac valves, and it extends fully outward, growing through the muscle sidewalls until there is a complete physical (and electrical) separation of the top and bottom chambers. At that early separation point in the womb, the upper atrial chambers will activate independently from the lower ventricular chambers, and the rhythmic, efficient co-ordination of blood flow is established.

Again, about one in three hundred babies has a heart in which a residual outer strand or strands is or are left connecting the atria to the ventricles. Ironically, these little bands of muscle fiber were actually discovered and recorded circa 1899 (almost thirty years before WPW!) by a researcher named Stanley Kent. Kent performed detailed post-mortem dissections on numerous hearts, and didn't know what to make of these occasional little muscle straps. They became known as Kent Bundles, and were relegated to the archives of cardiac triviality. (Kent thought that they might even be normal structures that are just more pronounced in some instances.) Ultimately, Kent bundles are a miniscule structural defect *physically*; but they are *electrically* active and serve to carry normal electrical impulses over the side and (aberrantly) down into the ventricles ahead of schedule. Thus, we see the Delta wave jumping in briefly, preceding the much stronger QRS wave—which essentially blows the Delta wave out of the picture under normal circumstances. In the race to ventricles, the aberrant Delta wave gets a head start, but the much faster (His-perkinje) conduction of the QRS spike wins the race. (Normally, that is!) However, depending on the location of the Kent Bundle and the excited state of the cardiac muscle, the Delta wave can periodically undercut and overpower the normal sinus triggering of the QRS wave, by triggering its own, self-sustaining, reverse electrical flow pattern that goes down into the ventricle and back up through the central conduction fibers, back up into the atrial muscle again and over the side, down through the Kent bundle again, and back up through the atria—round and round, round and round—totally chaotic—triggering and whiplashing the heart muscle up to two hundred and fifty times a minute. This is the "active bout" of WPW. Eventually, the heart muscle fatigues (the repolarization lags) and the crazy Kent bundle "circus rhythm" or "re-entry rhythm" (as it is called) will stop on its own, and the normal p-(delta)-QRS rhythm returns, emerging out from under the electrical disturbance.

Briefly, in terms of medical treatment, for the vast majority of cases, there are atrial medications that can tone down the muscle, and prevent the emergence of these active bouts, but in a very few severe cases, surgery can be employed to go in, cut the Kent Bundle, and sever the electrical connection outright.

Clinically, in final bullet point summation:

If a person is born with a Kent bundle, they will have a Delta wave on their EKG, and they will be diagnosed as having WPW.

Not all people with a Delta wave get the bouts of tachycardia. Much depends on the location of the Kent bundle around (what is called) the Atrio-Ventricular ring.

Many people can go their whole lives not knowing they even have a Delta wave, if they never had an EKG. (I had a twenty-year-old male RT student in 1987 on whom we did an EKG, for academic purposes, in class. Lo and behold, he had a prominent Delta wave. He subsequently went to his doctor, and they resolved to keep an eye on it. Almost thirty years later, he's still working at a hospital in town, and he's never had an *active bout* of WPW.)

OK. You get the basic idea about WPW. It's a teeny congenital defect, with the potential to have a profound electrical effect on the heart. With that preliminary, clinical background in place, we now progress to the all-important refrigerator repair job. And just how does WPW clinically tie in to that? Thought we'd never get there.

In 1988, as a bachelor, I bought my first house, and it needed a new refrigerator. To minimize costs, I searched for used refrigerators in the classified ads in the newspaper: how Cro-Magnon is that? I found a beautiful double-door high-capacity unit for a hundred dollars; a new unit like that would probably have cost eight hundred or nine hundred dollars, at the time. I thought I had scored a major bargain. Unfortunately, after getting it home the refrigerator completely konked out a few days later. I got down underneath it, to inspect the refrigeration pump, etc., and it was all smothered by a dense mouse or rat nest of some kind. I tugged out a whole lot of shredded debris to finally expose the working elements. And, as I was soon to learn, the working elements were totally cooked. So, it was back to the Cro-Magnon classifieds again, this time looking for a refrigerator repair man. I found a guy in South Tacoma who was repairing refrigerators out of his garage. He sounded like a chipper guy over the phone, so I got my neighbor to help me load the heavy fridge on to the back of my pickup truck, and off I went.

    This refrigerator repairman was an awesome and friendly person who was currently down on his luck on two counts. One, he was a Boeing machinist who had been recently laid off after several years of steady employment. Always a tough thing to deal with. He was repairing refrigerators at home now, to help make ends meet, until he could be hired again by Boeing. And two, to make matters worse, as he explained with a heavy heart, just the day before, his wife had been diagnosed with a "serious congenital cardiac anomaly." He had been fretting about it, and wasn't sure how to process the bad news, but his wife was on medication for it, and more testing was scheduled, and he was trying to be optimistic.

I told him that I was a respiratory therapist and had worked with many heart patients in the past, and I gently inquired as to the nature of his wife's problem.

Shaking his head, he said, "Oh it's a horrible thing. It's called Wolff-Parkinson-White Syndrome. Just saying it gives me creeps."

My ears perked, and I asked him what the doctor had told him about it.

He said, "I asked the doctor to explain it to me, but he said it was very complicated, and probably over my head. And how can I argue with that? Congenital cardiac anomaly. I guess my wife has a grossly deformed heart muscle from birth. I don't know, maybe it will require a surgical reconstruction of her whole heart."

At this point I couldn't help but to step in and to give him my own spiel on the matter. I assured him that I was no doctor, but I did know a few things about WPW. I first asked if his wife was having bouts of tachycardia, and he said that she never had any issues before, but in the last week she had a couple bouts of heart racing in her chest and that's why they had gone to the doctor the day before.

Trying to assuage him somewhat, I explained that the spooky "congenital" element amounted to rather tiny muscle fibers that had the ability to create an electrical disturbance. Then I drew out on paper (like I did in class), the congenital Kent Bundle aspect, and showed him the bump wave and the rhythm, and assured him that it did not constitute a *gross, morphologic, deformity of the heart*. In fact, the congenital aspect is so structurally small it would be meaningless, if not for the electrical aspect. And I told him about my student from a year earlier who had WPW show up inadvertently, and he hadn't had a problem with it, yet. And it wasn't uncommon for people with Kent bundles never to have a bout of tachycardia. His wife was in her forties and hadn't previously had any problems, so her Kent bundle didn't appear to be a chronically troublesome one at this point. And she had already been prescribed the common calcium channel blockers that will suppress those episodes. All in all, I told him that the doctor's office should have never sent them home with the idea of the wife having a "grossly deformed heart." That was an unfortunate and unsettling over-characterization of the WPW syndrome. Perhaps it was all a misunderstanding.

He was pleased with the information I gave him, and then he finally progressed to diagnosing my own (WRS) Westinghouse Refrigerator Syndrome. And, unfortunately for me, my diagnosis was terminal; all of the critical refrigeration components needed to be replaced. Eventually he gave me an estimate of two hundred and twenty dollars, and said he would have it completed by the following afternoon.

When I returned the next evening, he was in great spirits. He said he and his wife had returned to the clinic in the morning with the information that I had given them, and the doctor agreed that "gross congenital deformity" did not fit the clinical picture at all, and he was sorry that that had been somehow miscommunicated. And it was likely that the wife would not have any further issues as long she responded well to the medication. So, their initial worries about cardiac deformities—including fears of future open heart surgeries to repair them—were put to rest.

In the end, he was so pleased to have this medical monkey off his back, that he gave me an enormous discount on the refrigerator repair. He told me that he wasn't charging me for labor, he would only charge for the Freon, and he would give me the new refrigeration pump at his wholesale cost. And the pump wasn't going to be the decent, standard pump that he originally intended to use, but he decided to install a high-end Tecumseh Pump that would last for decades. (I didn't know anything about Tecumseh pumps, but I gladly took his word for it.) In the end, the original estimate of two hundred and twenty dollars had shrunk to seventy-six dollars out of the door. A tremendous bargain. And it was all owing to a little, well-placed knowledge about WPW. So, I encourage my respiratory students at the community college to study hard, to enjoy learning things that are beyond the routine work, and who knows, maybe someday a little extra medical knowledge can get them a discounted refrigerator repair job, too!

In historical epilogue, the trans-Atlantic WPW team worked for the better part of a decade, and then World War Two broke out for five years, and then Europe and England rebuilt for years after the war. Ultimately, it wasn't until the mid-1950s that the retired doctors Wolff and White took a cruise ship to England, finally to meet retired Dr. Parkinson face to face for the first time.

Obstructive Sleep Apnea, American Cyanide, and the Downfall of Nazi Germany

All in a Day's Work for a Homecare RT.

Few paired topics can prickle the nape and tear at the heart so much as that of Nazi Germany and the chemical cyanide. This unspeakably gruesome combination brings to mind the most heinous acts of man's inhumanity to man ever perpetrated in our history. So much so, in fact, that if someone told you (in advance) that an elderly sleep apnea patient would share with you a riveting personal story about his encounters with Nazi Germany and the usage of cyanide, no doubt you would expect to hear a real-life episode from the Holocaust. After all, what other life experience could possibly comprise the gory combination of these two mutually chilling elements? But yet, more than ironically, this World War Two story turned out to be a real-life episode of true grit, hard work, and, ultimately, one of the great, down-home, behind-the-scenes American success stories, that was, in its own way, crucial to bringing Nazi Germany, finally, to its much-needed demise.

Before discussing the dramatic details relayed to me by this elderly gentleman, some preliminary academic background will be useful. For all aspiring respiratory therapy students (as for most all nursing and allied health students in general) one of the prerequisite core classes is chemistry. General Chemistry can be fascinating and intellectually enlightening, but it can also be incredibly tedious and boring, depending on the specific topic at hand, and also on your mood at the time! (I learned that I was never in the mood for electron orbitals and sub-orbitals. Gag me with a B-17 Bomber.)

However, all of us compatriots working in the medical care /hospital fields eventually become acquainted with myriad chemicals and medicines, and (as related in the story) one common bedside chemical used in wound cleaning and tracheostomy care is good old hydrogen peroxide, chemical formula H_2O_2. It is essentially an unstable, over-oxygenated water molecule. (H_2O + another O!) It breaks down to water and oxygen gas (O_2) in the presence of ambient light and heat (which is why it is stored in a dark bottle). When applied to a wound in open air, it fizzes and foams up rapidly, as the oxygen gas releases. On the larger scale, highly concentrated hydrogen peroxides (powerful fifty to sixty per cent solutions) are used by NASA as a rocket fuel oxidizer, and they are used by industrial pulp mills to bleach paper products. But OTC (over-the-counter) hydrogen peroxides are only about one to three per cent diluted solutions. They are not strong enough to damage human skin, or even the mucosa of the mouth, as it can be carefully used as an antiseptic mouthwash. But for a germ on the microscopic level, that "oxygen fizz" is no fun. It's deadly. Even aerobic germs that use oxygen themselves can be annihilated with a quick overdose of H_2O_2. Finally, even the body's own neutrophils (primary white blood cells that kill invading germs) will break apart as they attack the germ, and will release enzymes to destroy the germ's proteins—and they will also chemically create and release hydrogen peroxide directly on to the germ. Hydrogen peroxide is chemically tricky for human engineers to produce commercially, but our human bodies have been manufacturing it for internal germ-killing for millions of years!

More on H_2O_2 and the elderly man ahead.

The other critical chemical in the old man's story is the aforementioned compound, cyanide. In its basic form, cyanide is actually a very simple chemical molecule. The primary structure is one carbon atom (with four bonding points) linked to one nitrogen atom (with three bonding points.) The primary formula is x—CN. The x is the last open bonding point left over from the carbon atom. In its most basic forms, the open valence is usually filled in with one of three different elements having a single bonding point: hydrogen (H), sodium (Na) and potassium (K). Hence the three basic types of cyanide are: hydrogen cyanide (H—CN) a gas, sodium cyanide (Na—CN) a crystal powder, and potassium cyanide (K—CN), also a crystal powder. All forms are equally deadly poisonous, but they also have many interesting and practical uses in industrial chemistry.

As a notorious physiological poison, however, cyanide instantly shuts down the body's mitochondria (cell power generators) by blocking the critical cytochrome-coxygenase system. Like ball bearings being jammed deep into the meshing gear-works of a clock, cyanide molecules obliterate the body's Krebs-cycle physiology, and ATP (adenosine triphosphate) production snaps to a halt. No other chemical poison can kill you both as rapidly and as thoroughly. In the Nazi death camps (Auschwitz in particular), the gaseous hydrogen cyanide was used in the concentrated pellet form of Zyklon B. (The original German formulas of Zyklon A and B were developed as legitimate insecticides.) The two Nazi chemists —Bruno Tesch and Karl Weinbacher—who developed, canned and distributed the rapid-release, genocidal B formula to the extermination camps were themselves tried and executed for their heinous chemical engineering.

However, on the current, practical utilitarian front, every year thousands of tons of cyanide-based chemicals are used to make several types of modern polymer plastics, nylon fibers, and upholsteries like Naugahyde. From a gastro-intestinal standpoint, one could chew on and ingest such inert materials and not be affected by the bound cyanide components. But from a respiratory standpoint, when such common materials are burned in a fire, cyanide gases are often released. Hotel and theater fires involving large amounts of furniture and fabrics and carpets are particularly prone to cyanide gas production, and, many times, victims have died from rapid cyanide poisoning, before succumbing to either smoke inhalation or burns.

With this overview of related chemistry set in place, the central story begins.

In the course of my respiratory home care work years ago (circa 2003), certainly the topics of Nazi Germany and cyanide were the furthest things from my mind as I pulled up in front of the opulent, Bellevue-Washington-area home. The broad single-level home seemed to float on a raft of lush, colorful rhododendron bushes. Porting a couple of bags of CPAP equipment, I waded up the walkway between the bushes to the plantation-style porch. The front door to the home was over-large and already opened, and just inside, on the floor, a couple of workers on knee pads slid about, fitting new pieces of oak flooring into place.

Standing at the busy threshold, I was uncertain of how to navigate further, and then a woman standing well beyond the work crew signaled me to come in. I edged around and over the new flooring and stepped into an open cream-carpeted area with a raised dining room on the left and a sunken living room on the right. The woman introduced herself as the daughter-in-law of the man whom I was there to see, and she invited me to set my equipment bags on the broad wood dining table for the moment.

She was about to search for her father-in-law, but he appeared on his own, having just stepped out of the same work area through which I had come. He stood there at the edge of the carpet, slender, bent over on his cane, his puffy, button-up blue shirt and his baggy khaki slacks each appearing a size too large. His white hair was thin but well-groomed back, and his spectacles rested a little outward on his large, hawkish nose. The daughter introduced me as the respiratory therapist, and, even before he made his short response, I just had the stereotypical assumption that his voice would be somewhat raspy, even crotchety perhaps. But his resonant tone was unexpectedly smooth and baritone, intellectually reverberating (if there is such a thing.)

"Why, yes," he said graciously. "Nice to see you. Come follow me."

The elderly gentleman then led me back over the remodeled floor, beyond the workers, farther down the hallway and up to a bedroom door on the right. Inside, the bedroom was not cramped, but certainly smallish. Straight ahead was one window on the far wall with an office desk beneath it. There was a single bed in the right-hand corner, and a cushy recliner set forward in the left corner. He took a seat in the recliner, and I took the central office chair, using his desktop as my assembly area.

As I sat there, unpacking the CPAP equipment, I couldn't help but swivel my head (furtively I thought) at the three, large-framed pieces of artwork that dominated the small walls around me. The thick, Gothic frames were necessarily sturdy enough to secure the large plates of glass within them, but the large poster-like pictures themselves were not expensive prints or paintings of any kind. Oddly, they appeared to be giant aerial photographs of what seemed to be complex industrial areas. Having spied my distracted, inhibited interest in his personal gallery, he gently offered in his soothing voice, "those are all pictures of chemical factories."

At that point, briefly released from the business at hand, I swiveled my chair all the way around to take in a fuller view of these three chemical factories. Exuding the same affection that one might display when highlighting pictures of one's own children, he first pointed to the largest of the three pictures on the wall to our right and explained, "That big factory there is in Tennessee. It's actually several chemical factories, constructed in close proximity to each other." For the moment, it looked to me like a vast conglomeration of piping running amidst and between an uncountable number of round and tubular storage tanks and buildings. In the general center of the maze-work was the oldest section, with newer sections having been built outward around it. Under his tutelage, I was able to discern three distinctly large, bulbous tanks in the middle region that were submerged in the snake-work of pipes.

"Those are my three babies right there," he said proudly, reminiscent. He went on to explain. "After the war, there was a big commercial push to produce non-chlorinated bleaching and oxidizing agents. The best alternative to chlorine bleach is highly concentrated hydrogen peroxide. I'm a chemical engineer, and I developed, and eventually patented, three different industrial methods for mass-producing hydrogen peroxide. And that old factory section right there is still running strong and making hydrogen peroxide today."

He was not the original chemical producer of hydrogen peroxide, but his unique processes were the genesis of modern, high-yield production for both personal and industrial use. I was certainly impressed. How many of us have used over-the-counter hydrogen peroxide to clean infected cuts and so forth? We don't often get to meet or to know the individuals who pioneered such common household items. Pointing then to the second picture, he went on to explain other chemical projects and even chemical capers that he and his young lab mates had perpetrated. In one particular chemistry project, he had had occasion to work with pure sodium, which is highly combustible if it contacts water. Just tossing a small chunk of soft, sodium metal into a water bath will set off a sizzling, flashing fireworks show—apparently much to the surprise of passers-by along the company campus pond, who subsequently went running for their lives, as the chemical imps in the bushes snickered.

But all elemental hijinks aside, the mood mellowed dramatically when the topic of the third picture came into focus. It was the least impressive of the three facilities, at least from a complex aerial standpoint. It was smaller in stature, with not nearly the same number of sprawling buildings, nor the same density of piping. But it was obvious by his demeanor that this chemical factory held a special place in his heart over and above the other two. He began by pointing out that the building of this factory was the first major chemical engineering project of his career, right out of college, in the heated build-up to World War Two. As a matter of national security, in response to an embargo imposed by Hitler, this critical factory was devoted to producing the *three variants* (hydrogen, sodium and potassium) of the primary chemical, cyanide. It was America's first industrial-scale, high-yield cyanide plant, and it was (at the time) located in the desert outside Riverside, California.

At this juncture, I was definitely intrigued by it all: Riverside, cyanide, California, Hitler, World War Two. This peculiar plot thickened by the second. I had never heard of anything like this before. Somehow, in the grander scheme of historical things, we had the early land of the Beach Boys standing up to the Third Reich by way of chemistry nerds fresh out of school. And somehow the whole imbroglio was centered on cyanide? My mind buzzed with questions: What made American cyanide so critical at the time? What embargo did Hitler impose? Why Riverside, California? What was the larger connection to Nazi Germany?

Odd though it all seemed, the scenario fell into place quickly, as the old man explained it. The critical nexus of it all was *metal plating*. Specifically, silver plating. Still another aspect of cyanide chemistry is that it is critical to the industrial process of silver-plating high-stress engine parts. More specifically to the time, potassium cyanide and silver plating were absolutely essential to the aircraft assembly lines building the Merlin engines for the P-51 Mustangs, the Hellcat engines for the aircraft of the US Navy, and Boeing's bomber planes, among several others. Without the silver plating to crankshaft and piston connections and associated bearings, the engine parts would not hold up to the high stress and heat created by these advanced, piston-driven power plants. Underlying and undercutting this reality was that nearly all the industrial cyanide in the world at the time was produced in Germany. The prowess of German engineering held serve in many industrial sectors at the time (aircraft, automobiles, rockets and so forth), but in none more so than in chemical engineering. German chemical factories were so far ahead of the rest of the world that it was far cheaper (pennies on the dollar) to import German chemicals than to produce them domestically. As things came to a head in the air battle over Britain, and as the U.S. was successful in re-supplying aircraft to the embattled British, Hitler cut off all chemical exports to America and the allied countries. Even though the Nazis hadn't declared war on America yet (and would not for another year and a half), the old man lamented that this was something that the U.S. should have prepared for a whole lot earlier, but so be it. All of a sudden, with an inadequate domestic production and a dwindling imported stockpile, the American and Allied war effort needed a cyanide boost, and needed it now!

The old man sighed, and then he reminisced purposefully, patriotically. Like the first few chugs of steam from a train leaving the station, he extolled the virtue of what talented human beings can accomplish when they put their minds to it. It still amazed him after all these years how well this entire project emerged and blended together on so many technical fronts at once. First, they needed a remote location to produce the chemical, but near enough to a seaport for rapid exportation. They also needed a dedicated rail line to bring the raw materials in, and then safely to take the finished product to the newly built port facility. Enter Riverside, California. It had a remote desert to the east, but was near enough to the port terminals of Los Angeles to the west.

The momentum of the old man's words steamed ahead, faster and smoother. His mellifluous voice was now roaring down the tracks. He recalled the grandeur of seeing all those teams of good men hard at work. They were men with a mission, and their determination abounded in the relentless sounds of tools and machinery, all coordinated to one collective purpose. He spoke of the thrill of seeing his own blueprinted handiwork rise up for real off the desert floor. At the same time, miles away, with equal vigor, the port facility was rising up off the beach, even as huge tanker ships already waited at anchor offshore, eager to load and to transport the first shipments. In between both locations, night and day, rail crews urgently put the lines in place. Like impatient leviathans, locomotives, trailing long loads of chemical cars and equipment, constantly nosed into the work area, inching forward as each track section was dutifully laid down in front. Time was of the essence, and every worker knew what was at stake. For him personally, it was a spectacular process to behold and to be a part of, and, in the end, the factory blazed into life, the trains rolled, the ships sailed, and the critical product was delivered in time. It was down to the wire, but American and British aircraft production continued without interruption. And ultimately, so too did the demise of the Nazi Empire.

And that's when this mellifluous, mild-mannered, man, eighty years old or so, lifted his cane, brandished it at the picture and said, forcefully, "Hitler and his scientists thought they had American scientists over a barrel. But we showed them. They messed with the wrong people. We whipped their Nazi fannies!"

Quite an incredible and uplifting story to say the least. And as the bravado slowly faded in the aftermath, the old man gingerly added his own personal epilogue to the timetable. After the cyanide project, it was immediately after the war that he got involved with the hydrogen peroxide development, and I recalled him mentioning that he held three patents in that regard. I asked him if he got compensated for his patents, and the answer was "yes and no." As a company employee—and the company was either Dow or Dupont, I forget which—the patents were essentially shared, but the bulk of control was retained by the corporation. By and large, his name was on each patent and that was about it. However, he wasn't complaining. The company did give him some generous bonuses, and since he was a single man at the time, he had enough money to buy his own Piper-cub style airplane. And in the latter nineteen-forties, he had spent the last couple of years of his bachelorhood taking extended barnstorming trips with fellow pilots. He talked about the sheer joy of cruising over the farm fields and the church steeples of rural America. Pastures and ponds, painted barns and silos, cows and horses, rivers and lakes—he got to see rustic rural America at the height of rustic rural America. And all from above. Also, he said a popular tactic for barnstormers back then was to land at county fairs and offer rides, free to children and a couple of bucks for adults. It was a good way to pick up some quick gas money. At this point I couldn't help but to see this part of the episode as an erstwhile collusion of *'Illusions* and chemistry.'* It was something on the order of "Richard Bach meets the Periodic Chart of the Elements."

(The barnstorming, metaphysical novel *Illusions* by Richard Bach is an uplifting and inspiring story, as well.) And, yes, the old man did in fact read that book, too. It reminded him of his youth.

When my homecare business with him was concluded, I shook his hand and told him how much I had appreciated his story. It was a wonderful recitation to hear, and it surely spoke to the human grandeur of another time and another place. Presently, as America's greatest generation fades into the past more quickly than ever, it's important to remember the contributions of everyone in that era—and not just of those who fought on the battlefield, but of those who contributed at home as well. Not to be too critical of today's youth, but, in comparison, there is a vast developmental gulf between the nineteen-year-olds of today and those of the greatest generation who actually flew the missions in Europe. The perspective can be summed up by the colossal difference between a person playing an air-war video game at night in bed, and a person actually flying a real B-17 at night against real flak and real German fighters in a bombing run over Schweinfurt—two-thirds of whom never came back. And to add a retro-active dimension, all the brave young men who did made it back from those nightmare flights, flew on engines with silver-plated parts that kept them airborne long enough to get home. It's impossible to comprehend the total number of contributions and sacrifices made by American people to the cause of World War Two. But each time a new perspective is realized it is important to acknowledge it and to appreciate it.

As I got into my car outside, I could see the old man's bedroom window peeking above the rhododendron bushes near the far end of the house. It was a nice place to be, all things considered. Being both surrounded by family in your twilight years, and living in a room surrounded by your own most intimate accomplishments, is something to be wished for all. I felt very fortunate to have met this man and to share his story. At the same time, I couldn't help but wonder how many bedroom windows we pass in our daily travels, never knowing the trials, tribulations and inspiring stories of the occupants within. All along the bottom of our ocean of air, there are so many windows, so little access, and so, so little time.

Consequently, I have found such golden opportunities to be one of the ineluctable amenities of modern respiratory home care.

Microsoft Windows (Obstructive) Sleep (Apnea) Mode and Other Off-Campus CPAP Adventures

Consider the following question: do nerds get sleep apnea? It is not a very compelling question, by modern medical standards, but it does have a profoundly definitive answer: yes. Nerds do get sleep apnea. And since I have some past experience setting up Microsoft employees on CPAP systems at their Redmond, WA facilities, I am not just a witness to the fact, but I am a first-hand perpetrator of aiding and abetting nerds with their sleep apnea equipment. And I learned that, up close, a lot of nerds don't even look like nerds most of the time. But all told, one can learn a lot of fascinating things about science, computers and software development by just a spending a little time with those who do this high-tech stuff for a living. And, in the end, as a respiratory clinician, I gained a helpful perspective for encouraging reluctant sleep apnea patients to persevere with their CPAP treatment and compliance.

Again, one of the major amenities of working in respiratory home care is that you get to meet and to interact with so many different people. And you don't always meet them either in the clinic office or at home. Adding even more interest to the interactions at times, not infrequently, schedules depending, arrangements are made to set up equipment in a confidential location at the person's workplace. Getting to absorb the sights, sounds and personal dynamics of someone else's work environment, in real time, is something not many of us get a chance to do. In that regard, I have set up CPAP equipment in such places as a factory that manufactured ornate, decorative wind chimes (it was a colorful and tingling experience). On two occasions, I have set up equipment at dairy farms. One was a small family farm, and the other a large regional dairy corporation. I learned some amazing things at each location. If you have ever sat at a stoplight, trundling your fingers on the steering wheel, intensely pondering whatever happens to all that grain mash that is routinely discarded by beer brewers and distillers, well, I can finally assuage your curiosity with the answer: dairy cows eat it and convert it to milk. The family farm had a contract with several local brewers to have the mash routinely dumped into huge bins on site. It gave the brewers a free place in which to dump their unusable by-products, and it gave the cows a free and nutritious food supply. (Maybe even a little buzz!) Amazingly, the distiller's mash goes from making brewski to making mooski. Who'da thunk it?

Likewise, the corporate dairy farm had a similar industrial connection that reached all the way to the Philippines. Only this enterprise involved eggs. Aside from their huge milk production facilities, this dairy also had many acres of chicken houses. They packed and sold eggs the standard way, in cartons, but, on a much larger scale they also had gigantic automatic egg-cracking and bagging machines that generated thousands of pounds of egg shells per year. Is there a market for broken, discarded egg shells? Absolutely. Feeding ground up egg shells to baby shrimp dramatically increases their calcium intake, and accelerates their growth rate. Shrimp farmers in the Philippines are happy to pay good money for egg shells in bulk.

Another time, I did a CPAP set up in an office perched above the factory floor of the Genie Lift Corporation—a fastidiously clean, brightly enameled work environment, with a Ping-Pong table, and multiple game units in the center of the factory floor, for the employees to use at break time. One would typically expect a factory that manufactures numerous, large, motorized hydraulic contraptions to be a dutifully greasy and grimy environment. Not even. The Genie factory is a sparkling operation, and from the look I got at it, a cheerful and fun place to work. According to the supervisor whom I was there to see, the whole, super-efficient, spotless layout was tailored after the *Toyota Company Model*. Each day, the tools and the exact number of parts and pieces for assembly—down to the individual nuts and washers—are pre-positioned for each worker's station. There is no fishing for parts or pieces, or doubling back to a tool rack for a different wrench, etc. Each worker shows up at their station, they have at it for the shift, and then they head home. No muss, no fuss, no wasted time.

Regarding Microsoft now, in the early 2000's, I worked for a respiratory homecare company in Tacoma that, as a course of downsizing, had to close its satellite branch in Kirkland, WA. Subsequently, I was assigned to cover that large northern sector from out of our Tacoma branch. Consequently, I spent many hours in creeping traffic on the S.R 167 and I-405 corridors. For all those bumper-to-bumper compatriots who can relate to this autobahn of the damned, try negotiating it for a whole summer in an old Nissan Sentra with a broken air conditioner. From Sumner to Bothell it was hell on wheels, and very slowly-turning wheels at that. But anyway, from Tacoma we still serviced many referral sources in the Bellevue-Redmond area, and many of those doctors' offices serviced Microsoft employees. And I remember well the first CPAP set up that I did on the Microsoft main campus. The client was a young woman, and she instructed me to meet her (if twelve-plus-year-old memory serves me correctly) in Building Nineteen.

 I was excited to get to go on the Microsoft campus and to see the inside of one of the buildings. Not being the least bit cyber-savvy myself, I have always had thorough admiration for those gifted humans who can comprehend such things as programming a computer to play chess, or to create the endlessly interactive cells of an Excel sheet. It totally boggles my pre-analog mind. Anyway, for some reason, I was expecting to see complex laboratory rooms teeming with nerds in white smocks, working on leviathan gut piles of tangled-up wires, diodes and circuit boards, maybe even using micro-soldering tools that gave off sparks. But a Star Wars repair garage proved to be the furthest thing from a Microsoft facility as there could be. Relating to other return trips as well, the buildings I went inside of were all but identical in style and layout. The hallways were long, the office doors were taller than average, and after passing so many office doors a snack-bar vending-service alcove would emerge. Like binary digits, this staccato pattern repeated itself—office rooms and snacking locations at precise intervals. I was curious. And just what the heck was it that took place in these buildings that spurred the generation of global globzillions of dollars? Well, I was about to learn.

The lady (software developer) whom I had come to meet took me to the end of one of the hallways, to a small waiting area, and we performed the CPAP set-up there. It wasn't a totally confidential location, but local foot traffic was exceedingly sparse. (And I suppose there also exists an axiomatic *nerd's creed* that what happens at Microsoft, stays at Microsoft.) In the course of our therapeutic interaction, I had occasion to inquire about the office building layout, the nature of the work she did there, and so forth. For her own sensibilities, with a considerable economy of words, she summed up my general questions in a single word: "Help."

"Help?" I repeated.

She nodded and explained that all the operations in this building were devoted to the HELP functions in all Windows programs. Anywhere and everywhere in Windows Applications that you find a HELP option / dropdown box, it is overseen by the developers in this building. And all those HELP functions need to be relentlessly updated and rewritten, as newer software applications are brought on board.

That all made instant sense. Just looking at MS Word, there are numerous independent functions on the tool and task bars, and logic would suggest that someone had to oversee developing and updating them. In Microsoft world, it may not take a village, but it does in many cases take a whole building to stay on task. Then I asked about the workplace environment. I admitted that I had perhaps naïve visions of cyber labs and high-tech gizmos (maybe even R2-D2 walking his bionic pet ferret down the hall on a laser leash), but most of this seemed like regular business office space, with ample snack bars available. Well, there was a method to the mundaneness as well. She explained that the clear majority of time spent in software development is in talking with (and yes casually snacking with) the users of particular software. Businesses, schools, colleges, insurance companies, and so on: it is the interested parties who actively use the software who come up with suggestions on how to expand the functions of the programs, better to aid their businesses. It takes a lot of verbal interaction to distill down exactly what the issues are and, ultimately, what the subsequent software development would need to accomplish. This is how the real world influences the software world and back again.

Regarding the *ultra-high-tech* stuff (the micro nuts and bolts), eventually, this information can wend its way down to the actual microchip level in terms of enhancing the hardware to accommodate the software. That's where it gets real *geekazoid to the max*, and there are other buildings (and even other companies) that take care of that. She told me that she has observed microchip engineers walking on a twenty-foot by twenty-foot, millions-times-magnified picture of a microchip. At that extraordinary magnification, all the microscopic interconnections can be clearly seen, and the engineers can plot different strategies on how, ultimately, to make the microchips do what the end-user customer would like them to do. Fascinating. One can only marvel at the Byzantine processes that result in the on-screen conveniences and entertainment features that we take for granted.

And now, years later, looking back, in lieu of more recent futuristic development on the respiratory homecare front, all the newest CPAP machines have internal transmitting hardware and software that can relay detailed reports of sleep data to a secure cloud site, where doctors' offices and homecare companies can review it. CPAP patients themselves can join the web sites and track their own data reports on their PC, or have data report summaries sent directly to their smart phones (i.e., how many hours did you sleep last night? How many times did you stop breathing—and was it an obstructive apnea in the throat, or a central apnea in the brain? How often, and to what liter-flow, did your mask leak? And so forth.) Ironically, none of this latest, detailed, flashy CPAP technology was available twelve years ago, when I was servicing the Microsoft campus! (Who knows? Maybe I could have impressed *Microsoft employees* with my own cyberwares!)

And speaking of impressive, this next, concluding story of a Microsoft CPAP patient is fascinating from a corporate business and operations perspective. I set up this sleep apnea client in his office on the Microsoft West Campus on the other side of HWY 520. The West campus had the same general buildings, but was much cozier than the main campus. The buildings encircled a central courtyard that included a company cafeteria. Trust me, in Microsoft world, the pedestrian word *cafeteria* actually translates into *spectacular dining plaza*. There was a massive salad bar, a burger bar, a Chinese food bar, a Mexican food bar, Italian pizza bar...Anyway, I had a wonderful lunch there that day with the CPAP client, and believe me, if I worked for Microsoft, I would be far more overweight than I currently am.

On topic, this CPAP client was employed as a technical writer. A highly accomplished word geek, he was a lapidary, skilled in the cleaving and polishing of verbal gems. Less eloquently, he was a linguistic gardener who often had to take a cerebral weed-whacker to verbose and gangly company copy. And, as he happily related to me during our lunch that day, his very first writing project as a Microsoft employee had proved immensely satisfying.

To begin with, he was originally from the Midwest (the Wolverine State, as I recall) and right out of college he had secured a well-paying job as a technical writer back there for another local software developer. But as far as he was concerned, be it ever so local, and even well-paying, it did not in any way carry the upstanding reputation of working for Microsoft. He didn't just covet the prestige of working for Microsoft, he craved it no end. His unbending goal was to get hired by Microsoft and to move to the Seattle area and to work there for his entire career. Veni, vidi, vinci. Done. Finito. Not interested in any other alternative.

In fact, he was so determined to work at Microsoft that he spent over two years submitting and resubmitting applications and resumes. Upon each rejection, he would immediately re-write them and resubmit them again. (He kept clicking his heels and repeating, *there is no place like Microsoft, there is no place like Microsoft.*) At long last, his laborious persistence finally paid off. Microsoft contacted him for an interview, so he flew out to Seattle immediately and eagerly went through the interview process, and, to his great pride and joy they hired him! It was the sentinel moment in his working life.

As a newbie tech writer, he had never met the two celebrated owners of the company, nor did he expect to any time soon. But early on, a writing project came down from on high, and it was assigned to him; it involved the global technical support call line. At the time, anyone calling the Microsoft technical support line would get an initial ninety seconds of explanation and routing choices. This recorded message was now deemed to be excessively long, perhaps tedious, and evidence revealed that many callers hung up before getting the complete information. Not good. The task (the mission—and he had to accept it!) was to laser-cut this verbosity down to less than half the time (thirty or forty seconds, max) while still retaining all the essential information of the original recorded message.

It seemed like a mighty tall order, but he buckled down and went to work on it right away. And down deep he knew he was going to do an exemplary job. After all, how could he not? Newbie aside, he wasn't just any technical writer. He was a Microsoft technical writer. And that meant something. He was a no-clichés-taken-prisoner, cyber-linguistic bad dude if there ever was one. Admittedly, he said that he darn near drove himself crazy with all the re-writing, but he kept plugging away at it, and he was cautiously confident at the finish. He submitted the completed project to the powers that be, and he kept his fingers crossed.

Soon thereafter, he was scheduled to make an appearance at an executive meeting where his project was a brief item on the agenda. When he joined the meeting in progress (knees trembling) he briefly got to see the celebrated founders at first hand. When his project came up, it was read aloud and the assembled committee approved it unanimously, with much kudos. The new global tech line recording was a definite go. The committee thanked him for a great job, and he said that he left that meeting absolutely euphoric. He was in a state of near levitation. All those years of submitting and re-submitting resumes had just paid off, in spades! He had got the job done, and had made a solid impression, in front of the entire executive leadership. What new employee could ask for anything more at Microsoft? Or any other company for that matter?

Feeling oh-so good, oh-so fine, he said that he strutted out to his car in the parking lot, fired up that engine, and started to drive out toward the highway to go home and to celebrate his well-earned success. But then he slowed down and stopped. He briefly pulled his car back into a parking place again. Thinking about it, just for posterity's sake, he wanted to listen to the old ninety-second recording again. Maybe just to wish it a solemn goodbye. He pulled out his cell phone, dialed the Microsoft global tech number and, much to his surprise, his new forty-second replacement was already up and running. Worldwide! That fast! Really? Are you kidding me?

    He was stunned. He couldn't believe it. But then he had to remind himself. That's right. I work for Microsoft.

    All told, sleep apnea affects at least four per cent, and maybe even up to ten per cent of the population, high-end nerds included. In fact, no one is excluded. Obstructive sleep apnea used to be regarded as a mostly male, overweight, over-forty- years-of-age type of problem. But accumulated testing over the years had revealed that it afflicts all demographics, including young children. Lack of sleep throws all your body systems out of kilter, and the degree to which untreated sleep apnea disastrously compounds heart disease and stroke is an ugly topic for another writing.

    But the final takeaway here involves a common scenario for many sleep apnea victims. Often it is the spouse or partner of the victim who notices the breathing lapses and gasping at night, and often the oblivious victim doesn't want to deal with it. The initial road to the treatment of Sleep Apnea is often strewn with self-made roadblocks and delaying obstacles, and some couples endure years of arguing about it. In the meantime neither partner is sleeping well. For many, the thought of wearing a pressure mask connected to a hose at night is just too awkward and cumbersome even to contemplate. Who wants to wear a stupid contraption like that?

Well, perhaps, as an ameliorating tactic, it can be pointed out to the obstinate Sleep Apnea Sufferer, that some of the most intelligent people in this country do wear this stupid thing, and with great results. Often people find that CPAP isn't nearly the encumbrance it seems to be ahead of time. You only wear it while you sleep, and once the body adjusts to it, it's like it isn't even there. So, if you exhibit signs and symptoms of sleep apnea, and those closest to you are deeply concerned and want you to do something about it, do the wise thing and get it checked out. Be smart. Take command of your health care destiny. Ultimately, do as they do at Microsoft! Unleash your inner nerd! *Control-Alt-Delete* all running procrastination programs. *Minimize* the EGO page. *Defrag* all accumulated fears to one remote manageable location. *Maximize* the Family Matters page, and give it your best effort. You'll sleep better at night if you do. And your family will love you even more for it.

Happy Endings. The Complex Sleep Apnea Gremlin, the Distraught Lawyer, the Angry Judge and the Triumphant Gremlin Busters

Obstructive Sleep Apnea (OSA) is caused by soft tissue occluding the upper airway at night during sleep. The tongue and soft palate are the primary culprits, with other structures like tonsils, adenoids, and uvula contributing. Obstructive breath stoppages in the throat happen to everyone once in a while in their sleep, but in a significant percentage of the population (four to ten per cent) it happens so often that it becomes life threatening and requires treatment (most commonly, CPAP treatment). Ultimately, as observed and documented in a sleep study, in an active OSA event the diaphragm and chest muscles continue to struggle to breathe, but no breath is pulled in, due to the clogged throat. Eventually, the oxygen-starved body briefly wakes up, takes a big throat-opening breath, and then goes right back to sleep (and nearly always with no memory of the awakening.) And this miserable cycle repeats itself, many times per hour. Such is the observed, diagnostic process of OSA.

Concurrently, there is another manifestation of breath stoppage during sleep, called Central Sleep Apnea (or

CSA). In these events the throat is clear and open, and it is the brain (or central nervous system) that briefly stops sending nerve impulses altogether. The body lies there *not* breathing, with the diaphragm and chest muscles completely motionless, not even trying. As with OSA, the oxygen-starvation and carbon dioxide build up eventually become overwhelming and the body abruptly awakens with a gasp, and breathing resumes again. CSA is more complex and mysterious than OSA, but the graphic differences between them are simple and obvious to most any observer. In a sleep study report (polysomnogram – translated *many sleep graphs*), the OSA pattern shows a flat breathing line, and just beneath are the diaphragm and muscle activity lines, which are both frantically tracing their frustrated activity: no breathing—but muscles trying! In the CSA pattern, all three lines are flat: there is no breathing at all and no muscle activity at all. Because the airway is open at the time, CSA events are also nicknamed "clear airway apneas." Such is the straightforward, diagnostic difference between OSA and CSA.

However, this rather straightforward pattern of CSA can further manifest in a much more complex and paradoxical form of CSA called Complex Sleep Disordered Breathing (CSDB). The starkly paradoxical aspect is that this often-ferocious (Gremlin) form of Central Sleep Apnea can be unleashed by the very CPAP that is trying to treat the Obstructive Sleep Apnea.

Sounds strange, but here is the paradoxical Gremlin in a simplified sequence. A person has OSA. CPAP pressure is applied to fix the OSA in the throat. The person subsequently develops not just copious CSA events, but often even more dynamic central events called Cheyne-Stokes Respirations (CSR)—a periodic waxing and waning between hyperventilation and apnea and back again. In this case, the CPAP doesn't make the patient feel better, it makes the problem much worse. Take away the CPAP pressure from the throat, and the Central Nervous chaos subsides (the Gremlin retreats underground), but now the Obstructive Sleep Apnea re-emerges. untreated. CSDB is a perplexing neuro-pulmonary pickle to say the least. Luckily (on a couple of counts), this Gremlin form of Sleep Apnea is relatively rare (it only happens to about four in every hundred CPAP patients), and it can now be effectively treated with a more advanced BiPAP/Auto-Servo Ventilation therapy (ASV).

This advanced machine tracks the patient's breathing pattern breath by breath, and can make rapid flow changes as needed. It initially attempts to operate as a basic CPAP machine for OSA in the throat. But if a Central Apnea event occurs, the ASV machine will immediately step in and breathe for the patient, and then it will back away when the patient's own breathing returns. (ASV is somewhat of a "whack a Gremlin" mode.) And if the more chaotic CSR Gremlin emerges (fast breathing—slow breathing—no breathing—and back again), the machine will rapidly increase flow requirements for the smaller fading breaths, and decrease flow on the larger hyperventilation breaths in an attempt to stabilize the pattern overall.

Diagnostically, sometimes CSDB is caught early during the initial sleep study in the lab; more often, it is caught down the road by CPAP monitoring in the home. Thanks to elaborate monitoring algorithms and cellular technology, the CSDB Gremlin that haunts the CPAP community at large can skulk, but it cannot hide. All updated CPAP machines can both track and differentiate OSA and CSA events, graphically record them for report, and send that report to a cloud-based monitoring program. For instance, if a person on a CPAP machine stops breathing for longer than ten seconds, the machine itself will recognize an apnea in progress, and then it will also send out a *pressure pulse signal* to check the throat. If the throat is clogged, it documents an obstructive event, and if the throat is wide open, it documents a central event. It will also record the undulating, chaotic patterns of Cheyne-Stokes respirations, if they occur. And all this information is transmitted daily and made available to specific Durable Medical Equipment (DME) clinicians and doctor's offices. Ultimately, the updated (very smart) CPAP machine will thoroughly document the presence of the CSDB Gremlin, but outside of alerting the patient and caregivers, it won't be able do anything about it. The fix involves upgrading the afflicted patient to the aforementioned ASV machine.

As it turns out, from an insurance reimbursement standpoint, the cost of a regular CPAP machine is a little north of a thousand dollars, while the cost of an ASV machine is often north of six thousand dollars!

Given that ASV units are so much more expensive than standard CPAP units, it is easy to appreciate why insurance providers have developed strict, pre-authorizing clinical criteria to cover them. The need for ASV must be thoroughly justified. And as a final note on that perspective—clinically, like the proverbial tourniquet—when an ASV machine is truly needed, it is needed badly and quickly.

As a real-world example, the following story chronicles the trials (literally) and tribulations of a CSDB patient with whom I worked some years ago, prior to routine, web-based monitoring. (In that time frame, the SD card was brought in to the office for manual downloading.) This episode highlights the importance of diagnosing and treating serious complex sleep disorders early on, before the affliction can actually ruin one's life and career.

The patient was an elderly woman with a sparkling British accent and calm intellectual demeanor. In her work, she was a highly specialized public defender who focused on certain sensitive legal cases, involving clients who were too incapacitated or too mentally afflicted to defend themselves before the law. Needless to say, it was an occupation that required full attention to process and detail. Recently she had found herself increasingly tired during the day, and had caught herself nodding off in court during session. This bothered her both physically and professionally, so she wisely decided that she needed to see her doctor about it. It wasn't normal for her to be so routinely unrested. Consequently, her doctor ordered a home sleep study, and she tested positive for moderate to severe OSA, with just a sprinkling of CSA tossed in. Soon thereafter she came unto my services and I set her up on a CPAP unit which she tolerated quite well at the set up session in my office.

Less than a week later she called back, literally in tears, lamenting how much worse she felt, and how she was nodding off in court more than ever before. It was so bad that the Judge had first warned her about it, and then, further, had had to reprimand her for it; she now fretted that her position as a public defender might be in jeopardy. I had her come into the office immediately, and we downloaded her machine and the CSDB and CSR was textbook rampant! She was one of the four-per-centers, in a very bad way. This brand of CPAP machine had a thorough primary report format that displayed the ugly numbers up front. But it also had a hidden (secondary) graphic wave report that expressly tracked the CSDB activity. The graphic wave report showed the tremendous extent of the complex chaos. It was Cheyne-Stokes Respirations to the max! If the report had come with background music, it would have been the Twilight Zone! The unmistakable tracks of the suffocating Gremlin were running wild! We contacted her doctor's office, faxed both reports over, and suggested a new sleep study at a facility, this time to do an ASV challenge. Thankfully, given the gravity of her situation, this all got resolved fairly quickly and it wasn't too long thereafter that she returned to get her ASV unit.

And wow, did it make a difference!

She called back just a couple of days later, ecstatic. It was a huge turn-around. (One of the more profound in my career.) Even though it had only been two days, she hadn't been this rested in a long while. A huge burden had been lifted off her back. She felt great, and had a whole new vigor for her daily schedule. She considered the ASV unit to be lifesaving and momentous. And for me, it was another case to relish the opportunity to help someone who had a serious *problem within a problem* and to see it through to a happy ending. Ultimately, many collaborative hands are in on these kinds of patient-care episodes, from the PCPs who refer, to the polysomnographic clinicians who test and diagnose, to the respiratory clinicians who directly set up the equipment and do the follow up—and, of course, to the manufacturers at large who continue to improve the technology and tools that allow clinicians to recognize pathological developments, and to take action accordingly. In the end, we are all on the same team, devoted to the same clinical end: to treat Obstructive Sleep Apnea sufferers. And on those fewer, miserable occasions when CSDB dares to rear its ugly head—who are you going to call? The ASV homecare providers! The Gremlin Busters!

No Horsing Around. CPAP Works! Attestations and Testimonials from (Eventually) Happy Sleep Apnea Patients

Over the years, I have fielded numerous testimonials from patients on their use of CPAP for the treatment of obstructive sleep apnea. Not surprisingly, many sleep apnea sufferers were negatively predisposed to the idea of wearing a pressure device on their face at night. But yet, many became positively surprised, even exhilarated by the beneficial results that they experienced. CPAP may not be for everyone, but it sure works well for a lot of people, even when they didn't expect it to work at all. As initial illustrations, the first two patient examples provide an extreme range, between one who was in active denial about his sleep apnea, and another who was passively, even tragically, oblivious to it.

In the first case, I set up a large male patient in the office; he was polite, but casually indifferent to the details of the session. I could tell (which was easy to do under the circumstances) that his heart just wasn't into this *CPAP thing* at all. He absorbed the information panned face, like a stoic little kid who was going to chew and swallow his spinach without changing expression. He wasn't curious, he didn't ask many questions and, at the end, I wished him well, and he nodded perfunctorily and walked out. Within the week, he walked back into the clinic office unannounced. It turned out that he had pressed his head into the bedpost while asleep, and had cracked the forehead piece on his CPAP mask. No problem, we could swap that simply enough. I took him in to a private fitting room for the moment and asked how everything was going. He held up and teetered his broken mask at me said with an honest chuckle, *"You know, I wasn't going to give you two cents for this CPAP machine working for me at all. But I had to try it, because my wife and doctor were really on my case, and I just got sick and tired of hearing about it. But wow, I was really surprised what a difference it made. The very first morning I woke up with it I knew right away that my head and body were different. For me, my mental alertness in the morning was the difference between a black-and-white TV and a color TV.* (Great analogy! I tucked that one away. I have related to it many times when setting up new patients on CPAP.) Suffice it to say, he was another CPAP doubter turned happy convert.

Another recent (touching? heartbreaking? intriguing? take your pick) example of CPAP success came from a thirty-one-year-old, single male client, who, ironically never knew that he had sleep apnea until a new girlfriend informed him of his spooky breath stoppages at night. However, concurrently, he had fully recognized that in the last couple of years he had been exceedingly tired all the time, had little energy to exercise, and napped a lot during the day. Succumbing to his own analytical sensibilities, he simply resigned himself to the unfortunate conclusion that he was *"just a lazy person!"* That was it, just lazy. Plain and simple. You hear stories about people who, for whatever reason, are just plain lazy and lethargic, and he had to face the music that he was one of them. How else could he explain it? And he had to admit to himself that he was thirty years old now (getting on in life), and he was not a teenager anymore, and this laziness was just a natural consequence of getting old. He decided to accept his languid fate and to not beat himself up about it. *OK, I am lazy. There are worse things to be.*

Well, thanks to the new girlfriend's caring observations and encouragement, he finally got himself checked out by his doctor. He was then referred to a pulmonologist for a sleep study, and then started on CPAP and the results were life-changing. His laggard laziness evaporated and he was both physically and psychologically rejuvenated. He said that over and above the physical revitalization, the biggest benefit for him was the thankful, self-esteem-rescuing realization that he wasn't just a lazy lunk after all! He was ailing from a real "medical" condition—a condition that was "fixable"—and he got it fixed! And life was good. What do you know? He wished he could have known about it and acted upon it a whole lot sooner.

Another patient who came to love CPAP was an outdoorsman whose family had, for years, tried to get him to go to the doctor to see about his atrociously loud snoring and choking. But he kept resisting. Over the years his thunderous snoring often kept the family awake at night, until they began to get used to it by default (as you would get used to living next to an airport). The family wondered what it would finally take to get him to go to the doctor, and the clincher finally came one time when they went camping at a State Park in an open tent area. They got there late at night, and the family found a vacant spot to quietly set up their tent, amid the half-dozen or so other tents. They went to sleep and the father snored so horrifically, that when they got up the next morning, all the tents around them were gone! They had the meadow all to themselves. (Good going dad! It's our private meadow now!) The father finally resigned himself to the fact that he had a problem. He figured that, if his snoring could clear out a public campground, maybe he should get it checked out. He did, and he loves his CPAP, and now the whole family can sleep well, even the neighbors.

One of my all-time favorite encounters with an ornery CPAP curmudgeon (who quickly became a gloriously happy advocate) involved a middle-aged gentleman who lived on a spectacular, emerald green horse ranch. Unenthusiastic, to say the least, he resisted coming to the office, so, at the doctor's request, I drove out to his home to do the CPAP set up. As I drove up the road, along the vast, horse-speckled property, I could see white rail fences stretching way out over broad waves of green grass that rolled out to the horizon. When I arrived at the ranch mansion at the end of the long driveway, his wife greeted me at the door. The mansion architecture itself was a modern rendition of a multi-angular horse barn, with large dormers dominating the roof. The plush interior was entirely bedecked in equestrian motifs. The deeply sunken living room was semi-encircled by half a dozen, chest-high wooden cabinets with large (dog-sized) carved wooden horses standing atop them. In the middle of the sunken living room where we performed the CPAP set up, we sat at a large, clear-glass slab of a coffee table, for which the shiny, skeletal table legs were comprised of bronzed horse reins. This was horse country. Inside and out. Turns out it was also crabby curmudgeon country, as I was about as well received by the husband as a house-calling, blood-letting leach therapist.

From the front door landing, the wife led me down into the living room, where the husband was already seated on the couch, alongside the glass table. A cushy chair had been placed opposite the couch for me, and the wife took a seat beside her husband. He was scowling at me the whole time, and, after I placed the equipment bags on the table, and before I could break the ice with my usual introduction—he groused, "I'm really not sure about this. I may just decide not to do this."

The wife leaned in and consoled him, reminding him what the doctor had told them. I then chimed in, informing him that the first three months are a trial period anyway, and there was no immediate rush to get compliant with it. He could take his time, wear it for just a short nap, or even just wear it and watch TV; it was all part of the acclimation process. Plus, we would experiment with different masks and nasal devices and he could pick the one he liked best (or disliked least.)

That seemed to assuage his negativity, for the moment, and we continued. But it wasn't long before he was grimacing and shaking his head again. He really didn't want to do this, and he was determined to invent an exit strategy on the fly. The wife tried to console him again, but he would have none of it. He impulsively decided that he wanted a word or two with his doctor, so he pulled out his cell phone and dialed up the medical office and spoke to the receptionist. The wife surreptitiously smirked and rolled her eyes at me, as if to lament, "Sorry, I wish you didn't have to go through this." Perhaps it was his affluent status or something, but the husband hit telephonic pay dirt quickly, as he had the doctor on the line in less than twenty seconds. (An astonishing feat where I come from.) The intense conversation rebounded between them for a while, and eventually the doctor got the better of it, and the husband relented, taciturn, brow furrowed, mandibles flexing. He would go ahead and try it (against his own better druthers). The gleeful wife rewardingly patted Mr. Grumpy on the arm.

Finally, the therapeutic coast seemed to be clear so we at last progressed with the major parts of the CPAP set up, including numerous mask-fit trials and pressure tests. In all, the usual one-hour set up time had stretched into a full two-hour episode. When I eventually drove away down the driveway, passing several curious horses suspiciously eyeballing me along the fence line, I concluded that this was a nice place to visit but I wouldn't want to make a regular habit of making CPAP house calls here.

Well, it was only three days later that the phone rang at my office in Tacoma and, lo and behold, it was the equestrian crank-meister himself. He needed to have a word with me. I wasn't certain where this requested exchange was going to go, but I said, "Sure, how can I help you?"

In summary, his dissertation was as follows: *As you could probably tell, I wasn't keen on doing this CPAP thing at all. I was just going through the motions to finally get my wife and doctor off my back about my snoring and what not. But I'll tell you, I am absolutely flabbergasted at how much better I feel. These last two days have been unreal. My energy level is just ridiculous. First of all, I never did any work with the horses in the evening after dinner. After dinner, I would crash on the couch. I might get up, I might not. Eventually I'd get up some time in the night to go to bathroom and then off to bed. Since using this machine, the last two nights after dinner I'm out in the barn until nine, ten, eleven at night, getting all kinds of work done that I never had time to do. It really feels like I'm on drugs or something! And yeah, I was dragging my fanny around here, always tired and down, and just figured that hey, that's just the way I am. I'm tired, I'm grumpy, and if you don't like it, tough. But it doesn't have to be that way. I just never knew how much energy I was deprived of. I am totally sold on CPAP. And believe it or not* (he said, with self-deprecating humor)*, so is my wife!*

Responding, I told him that it was a wonderful thing to hear and that I was really happy for him. I eagerly concurred that many people get into that sleep apnea rut and don't question it. Or, just as often, don't even know about it. The underlying rut becomes the bedraggled, default normal disposition. And it is tragic how many people trudge on through life not knowing any better about it. But it is always great to see CPAP change someone's life for the better, and he was certainly one of the most dynamic turn-arounds with whom I have had the pleasure to work.

In the end, there are far and away more people today living with undiagnosed sleep apnea than there are CPAP users. And all aversions to eventual CPAP use aside, just getting diagnosed is the initial problem within the problem. Nearly always, most people don't know they have a sleep apnea problem until they make it someone else's problem, most often a spouse. And circumstantially, (like the earlier thirty-one-year-old patient) those singles who live without partners can persist for decades without someone noticing their breathing lapses at night. Sometimes it is during a camping trip with friends or the sharing of a hotel room at a convention where a cohort can inform them of their snoring-choking-breath-stopping problem during sleep. Even then, without repeated follow-on encouragement, will the isolated sleep apnea sufferer act upon it? Often not, unfortunately. It ought to be axiomatic that friends don't let friends ignore their sleep apnea. But unless you are sleeping with your friends, they are never going to know it. It is the most common inherent conundrum that interferes with sleep apnea diagnosis. And then, of course, there is the follow-on obstacle course of CPAP compliance. This has a whole new set of conniptions to deal with. Few human medical conditions are as deeply beset with both diagnostic and therapeutic obstacles as is CPAP for sleep apnea. The whole process can be an exasperating undertaking. But if you can muster the gumption to push yourself through the entire rodeo, you are likely to find that CPAP really works. No horsing around!

A Short Primer on Children, Sleep Apnea, CPAP and the Preternatural Flight of REM Boy!

By itself, sleep is such a complex neurological and physiological phenomenon that exploring the mysteries of it should qualify as one of the top three, final human frontiers. And those top three are as follows: 1. Exploring the cosmic depth of outer space. 2. Exploring and mapping the deep unknown ocean bottom; and 3. Exploring what really goes on in the physiological depths of the brain and body during sleep.

The first two frontiers are probably much easier to explore!

And the third, final frontier is not at all confined to the human species alone. While the over-sized human brain may egotistically boast a vast evolutionary complexity that requires sleep in its various stages of depth and electrical wave activity, even a fruit fly exhibits different stages of sleep activity in its dinky little brain. The sleep stage process is so commonly mandatory among all living creatures that you could probably assert that whether or not there is other *intelligent* life in the universe, whatever level of living multicellular creature is out there—it probably sleeps. (Maybe, for levity's sake, I'll posit the grand, universal law of the couch potato: I sleep, therefore I am.)

Ultimately, on this planet, all living things need their sleep—bugs, lizards, bats—and human kids especially!

The longer that Obstructive Sleep Apnea has been researched and tested, the larger the afflicted population has become. Years ago, the vast bulk of the OSA population was overly relegated to mostly adult males, over forty, overweight, thick neck, big tongue and so forth. Today, that demographic certainly is a large part of the OSA population, but less so from a percentile basis, as many other demographics have joined in, so to speak. OSA is much more of an equal-opportunity affliction than once thought. And the most recent demographic of concern is children. Children are far less tolerant of minor sleep disturbances than adults. In terms of pure Apnea episodes (total flatline-not breathing-longer than ten seconds), adults can easily have up to five apnea events per hour, and still be asymptomatic, with an oxygen saturation that stays within decent limits (above ninety per cent). An adult with those numbers could not qualify for CPAP treatment under most insurance plans. However, a child having five apneas per hour is serious, even if there isn't a plunging oxygen saturation. The sleep disturbance alone can have lasting behavioral and physiologic effects throughout the day. Even one to two apneas per hour (which is diagnostically meaningless for the adult) can be significant for some kids. Kids especially need their undisturbed rest, and are vulnerable to a host of common maladies if they don't get it. The following citation from the American Sleep Apnea Association elucidates these concerns well.

Does your child snore? Does your child show other signs of disturbed sleep: long pauses in breathing, much tossing and turning in the bed, chronic mouth breathing during sleep, night sweats (owing to increased effort to breathe)? All these, and especially the snoring, are possible signs of sleep apnea, which is commoner among children than is generally recognized. It's estimated that one to four percent of children suffer from sleep apnea, many of them being between two and eight years old.

Furthermore, while there is a possibility that affected children will "grow out of" their sleep disorders, the evidence is steadily growing that untreated pediatric sleep disorders, including sleep apnea, can wreak a heavy toll while they persist. Studies have suggested that as many as twenty-five per cent of children diagnosed with attention-deficit hyperactivity disorder may actually have symptoms of obstructive sleep apnea, and that much of their learning difficulty and behavior problems can be the consequence of chronic fragmented sleep. Bed-wetting, sleep-walking, retarded growth, other hormonal and metabolic problems, even failure to thrive, can be related to sleep apnea. Some researchers have charted a specific impact of sleep disordered breathing on "executive functions" of the brain: cognitive flexibility, self-monitoring, planning, organization, and self-regulation of affect and arousal.

(American Sleep Apnea Association. Website; sleepapnea.org, 2017).

The potentially disastrous health consequences of untreated sleep apnea in children are plain to see. One of the major issues of sleep deprivation in OSA, for both kids and adults, is the lack of, or near absence of REM sleep (Rapid Eye Movement). The experience of the REM stage of sleep is associated with dreaming, but, from a neurological maintenance standpoint, many complex processes are occurring in REM that lend to restorative sleep and overall brain-body health. One key function is memory. It is believed that, during REM, the brain sorts out what goes into long term memory versus short term memory, and which things to discard from memory all together. As we move through time, distance and circumstance each day, our minds accumulate memory like so much lint on Velcro: the streets we drove down, the traffic lights we stopped at, the elevators we boarded, all the people we interacted with, etc. How much of this daily lint needs to be stored, how much can be erased, and how exactly is that process commandeered and enacted? Mighty mysterious stuff, but as days fade into weeks we remember fewer details of the past, except for important things. (I know that, in my own case, I am amazed, sometimes, at how often memorable past events become out of sequence in memory. I think I may have a REM Gremlin working in the file room with a chronologic disorder.) Also associated with REM sleep is a temporary, deep muscle paralysis, which lends to a physical restoration in the muscles themselves. If you ever suddenly woke from an intense nightmare and felt briefly paralyzed, you actually were! You came out of REM faster than the REM state could disengage the entire body. For a brief, frightening instant, you know how it feels to be paralyzed from the neck down! In the absence of quality REM sleep, memory is not properly processed, muscles aren't properly restored, and forgetfulness and irritability are probably the most common symptoms among adults, and, among children, the whole miserable list above comes into play.

I have worked in Respiratory Home Care since August, 2000, and over the last seventeen years, the number of pediatric patients has increased steadily. In fact, children advanced into the CPAP arena faster than the industry itself was prepared for it. Important as it is to treat children suffering from OSA, taking care of OSA kids with CPAP therapy and equipment has always been an awkward endeavor. To this day, CPAP manufacturers still consider CPAP machines to be an adult-appropriate device, and an "Off-Label Usage Waiver" must be signed by the parent at the time of setting up their child. The FDA has approved CPAP therapy for children seven years and older and over forty pounds in weight, but much younger children are routinely set up per doctor's prescription. And until recently, for many years, there were no designated "children's sizes" of CPAP masks. Often the Extra-Small Adult full-face mask (covering the mouth and the nose) would fit an older kid's face, and a regular Adult Nasal Mask (covering the nose only) would work as a full-face mask on a smaller kid. But (nose-only) nasal masks are preferred for kids, and, thankfully, some adult designs came with a very small "petite"-size nasal cushion that would fit young children. Fitting kids for CPAP interfaces was a cobble-craft effort for many years. Currently there are a small handful of (cute and colorful) children's interfaces on the market, and I think that just two of them have FDA approval, which doesn't really mean anything. All's fair in love, war, and fitting kids with CPAP masks.

I have had so many enjoyable clinical experiences setting up cute little tikes on CPAP, it would be difficult to pick a favorite one. Granted, there were no small number of screamers and squirmers, who were determined not to wear a mask at all, but with patient parental assistance, even some of them eventually calmed down and managed to breath on the pressure mask OK. I have come to realize that, in many cases, making the CPAP set up a family affair helps a lot. Several times, I have set up young CPAP tikes, as their older and younger siblings looked on in curious amazement. Often, in these cases, the little boys tended to be stoic and taciturn, and determined to show the others what a little man they were. And the little girls tended to be more smiley and giggly about it, looking around and enjoying the rapt attention. And some further advice in that regard, for RTs and clinicians doing these CPAP set ups, is that when the tike is small enough to be in mom's lap, holding a teddy bear at the time, before even starting with the child, a good maneuver is to get a little pediatric oxygen mask for the teddy bear to wear first. The freebee O_2 mask will set your DME company back about thirty-seven cents, and it will be worth it, as your chances of successfully fitting the little person will increase greatly. For pediatric sleep medicine, I think it should be a mandatory part of the policy and procedure manual to always "treat the teddy bear first!" (or the Elmo, or Buzz Light Year...).

I'll finish up this pediatric venture with one of the more touching messages that I received from the parent of a

CPAP kid. I had set up a nine-year-old boy on CPAP at his home in the Graham-Kapowsin area one evening, and his mother relayed to me all the issues that had plagued him in recent years: Falling asleep in school, low energy at home, memory issues, irritability issues, and so forth. But since he wasn't a loud snorer at all (which the majority of OSA kids are) the prospect of sleep deprivation or sleep apnea wasn't immediately considered. They concentrated on a healthy diet, vitamin augmentation, physical exercise and so forth, but nothing seemed to work. So finally, just to rule it out, the family doctor ordered a sleep study in a laboratory setting (since home-sleep-study criteria for kids isn't established yet), and, lo and behold, OSA was diagnosed. I don't remember the actual number of apneas per hour, but I remember its being significant enough, even for an adult. The poor kid had had it rough for a very long time, but that was about to change dramatically.

Therapeutically, for all age groups, at all times (apnea sufferers or not), nothing but good comes from getting a good night's sleep. Everyone is cranky when they are unrested; digestion can be thrown off, important appointments can be forgotten, falling asleep at the wheel can happen! Getting regular and thorough mind-body rest can prevent a lot of damaging chuck holes from forming in your daily roadway. And one nice thing about CPAP is that, when it does work for OSA patients, the benefits are often felt immediately. (The chuckholes are suddenly not there anymore.) And for this little boy, the thrill he experienced, on top of the beneficial effects, was a memorable milestone for him. Within a couple of days of the CPAP's being set up, the mother called me to share a fascinating and touching moment that she had with her son. She hadn't given it much thought before, but, apparently, her son's chronic lack of REM sleep was so significant, that even after nine years of age, he had no concept of what "dreaming" was like. He had never dreamed before. Then she told me that in the morning he came rushing into her bedroom all excited—"Mom! Mom! I was flying all around by myself, high in the sky, and I crashed into the grass, but I didn't get killed! It was weird, and it scared my tummy, but it was fun!"

It's a fine and pleasant realization that CPAP therapy, as cumbersome as it can be at times, is still able to create such a wonderful, morning moment for a mother and her once-beleaguered son. Still another ineluctable amenity of respiratory home care.

- American Sleep Apnea Association, 641 S Street, NW, 3rd Floor Washington, DC 20001-5196

Telephone and Fax: 888-293-3650 email: asaa@sleepapnea.org

Copyright 2017. American Sleep Apnea Association, Sleeptember, A.W.A.K.E., are trademarks of the American Sleep Apnea Association.

Campomelic Dysplasia and a Beautiful but Abbreviated Childhood

The disease campomelic dysplasia is a heartbreaking genetic condition in which very few victims live beyond infancy. Colloquially, it could be regarded as a brutal form of dwarfism, compounded by severe skeletal softening and malformation. Those few who do survive into childhood are beset with a constellation of physical and developmental issues, primarily focused on incomplete facial and skeletal bone ossification and often severe respiratory issues due to erratic formation of the cartilage in the tracheal-bronchial tree. Leg and arm bones are poorly developed, often bowed, more flexible than stiff. And limb and hip joints are often not properly enjoined, and those small kids who can ambulate do so in a bow-legged, waddling manner. However, physical disability does not mean cognitive disability, and such was the case with the incredible little campomelic boy whom I was fortunate enough to meet and to take care of.

Circa 2004, the mother of the little boy informed me that campomelic dysplasia was extremely rare, and that, at that time, there was only one genetic institute in Europe that tracked it. Upon the birth of her son and the subsequent identification of it, she and her husband briefly flew to Europe (on the institute's dime) to donate some genetic samples for study. I had never heard of the disease at the time, but recently (in preparation for these essays) I have accessed many medical sites, and the current estimates are that CD occurs somewhere around one in one hundred and eleven thousand to two hundred thousand births. Still a wide range, very rare, but not fully nailed down. The next question, of course, is "how does one care for a child afflicted with CD?" Ironically, and luckily, the mother happened to a be a licensed practical nurse who worked for the children's hospital in Tacoma. And her husband was a highly mechanically inclined outdoorsman, with a camper trailer and boat, etc. It turned out that this little CD kid had landed in a highly capable environment. And I would venture to guess that his short, struggling, but happy life was one much fuller than average, under the circumstances.

I stepped into the respiratory homecare picture when the little boy was between four and five years old. Already he was as fully, functionally self-reliant as he could be. For the parents, the first two years after birth were the most difficult, as much respiratory and tracheostomy care was required. His airways were extremely narrowed, and were prone to clogging off with secretions. All newborns generally have a disproportionately large head relative to the lower larynx and throat structures in the neck. A young child with "croup" (a.k.a. laryngo-tracheo-bronchitis /epiglottitis), is a case in point. Croup, and its noted "seal-bark cough," is caused by the narrow tracheal lumen's almost swelling shut from internal inflammation. Also, structures like the epiglottis, immediately above, can swell over the top of the airway. In a cough, the restricted airway and/or the swollen epiglottis can vibrate like a fleshy, saxophone reed, launching off a shrill barking sound. Beyond three years of age, the lower trachea and airway structures proportionately enlarge, relative to the head and throat above, and, at that point, the risk of the tissue's swelling over the airway is greatly reduced, and the child has effectively outgrown the croup stage. In the CD boy's case, his airway was permanently narrowed, and he would suffocate if it hadn't been for the highly-specialized tracheostomy tube that was inserted in his neck below the larynx. But again, as he grew larger, it was less difficult to keep the airway from clogging. Furthermore, again, as he got older he was trained to do as much of his own care as possible. By age four, it was astonishing how well-trained in his own care this little guy was. The parents had done an exemplary job in helping this boy become an independently-functioning human being, under some mighty difficult conditions.

Even though he had gangly IV infusion lines going into sites in his arm, and feeding tubes into the PEG line on his abdomen, he could move around OK, pushing his little plastic shopping cart that had the infusion bags hung on poles attached to the corners of the basket. There were times when the medicine and feeding tubes could be detached from his body for a while, and he was free to waddle around by himself away from the IV cart. But always available nearby was his CPAP machine with a trach-adaptor. The exhausting, noisy work of breathing through the narrow lumen of his trach tube was substantial, and required frequent respites. He knew when to say when, and even while watching cartoons with his siblings, or playing a video game, he would retreat from the action and go sit next to his small, living-room bed in the corner, and attach the CPAP tube to his own tracheostomy site. The CPAP pressure inflated his airway, and temporarily made inhalation a whole lot easier, giving his tired breathing muscles a much-needed "breather" of their own. And further still, amazingly, the CPAP inflation helped to bring up secretions, and he dutifully clicked on the suction machine next to the CPAP unit, and took care of that, too. He retrieved and opened a small infant suction catheter and attached it to the suction line, and then he would remove the CPAP coupler, and suction his own airway! Then, thus rejuvenated, he shut all the equipment off, neatly packed the tubing away, and waddled back into action with his siblings again.

    The first time I watched this brave and determined little tike in action, I was inspired! Inspired by him, and inspired by the family that had so diligently trained and taught him so much in such a short period. And that wasn't the half of it! Having had a tracheostomy in place his whole life, he had never learned to speak at all, but he could emote with a variety of grunts and throaty sounds that generally matched his grin or his scowl. But don't think for a second that he was inarticulate, because he was highly fluent in American Sign Language (ASL). If he was really irritated with you, he had ways of succinctly and directly expressing it. His brothers and sisters were all adept enough with sign language themselves thoroughly to communicate with him. He was by no means a stricken, passive, incommunicado island unto himself. For all practical purposes, he was just another striving kid in the family, one of the herd, who just needed frequent IV, CPAP and suction breaks.

But still, when it came to actual family outings, particularly camping and fishing in the remote outdoors, one would assume there had to be practical limits to including a kid with CD and all his vital paraphernalia. The CPAP and Suction machines required electricity, as well as the important IV infusion and feeding pumps. Well, no problem for the dad. All these critical items can be run off inverters, attached to a bank of three oversize 12V marine batteries, stacked and belted on a hand-truck with a safety cover over it. But don't these big 12 V batteries eventually require recharging themselves? Of course, and that's what gasoline-powered generators are all about.

When this family of five kids plus parents headed out of town in their long, Winnebago-style motor home, they towed a small box trailer packed with all the little boy's medical and electrical contraptions. Some people combat adversity better than others, and these impressive parents were beyond unconquerable. Via relentless parental commitment, nothing was going to stop this little guy from being an active part of the family anywhere, any time. Even on a boat.

I made monthly visits and more to this family's home for the better part of a year, and I enjoyed the clinical contact. This incredibly industrious family was a real adventure to be a part of. And then, the little boy's respiratory condition worsened somewhat, and the simple CPAP unit that had worked well for so long was deemed inadequate for his condition. His doctors wanted him to have a more elaborate (and highly expensive) mechanical ventilator for nightly usage and to use as needed during the day. We were a smaller regional DME company, and didn't currently carry those high-end ventilation units. But I lobbied hard for our company to get one anyway, figuring that stepping up for this family would put us in good standing with local pediatricians, and would make us even more of a go-to RT homecare company for complex cases. But it wasn't meant to be. Our company just couldn't reconcile the high expense on a one-off basis. Consequently, a national DME company who had the units in stock stepped in, and took over the little boy's ventilation care. I was heartbroken by it, but there was nothing I could do. It was just the law of the DME jungle.

 Several months later, I was inside Mary Bridge Children's Hospital on some other pediatric home care business, when I ran into the little CD boy's mother in the hallway. We were surprised to see each other and we did a friendly embrace and she asked if I would like to see her son again. Of course! Absolutely! She explained that he had had a bout of pneumonia recently, and had been admitted to the hospital for the last several days, but he was doing better and they should be heading home in the next day or so. She led me back down the hallway to his room, and, as I entered, the little boy was sitting up in bed, legs crossed beneath the blankets, holding a video game controller in his lap.

 He looked up and saw me and gave me a happy grunt-squeal, and lifted his hand up, and I shook it and gave him a quick hug. He then returned to the important business of the video game with which he was grappling. My own son's all-time favorite, it was Sonic the Hedgehog and his little tag-along compatriot, Tails. In this case, they were struggling to avoid both obstacles and waterfalls, and when Sonic got hit, the accumulated rings would splatter in jingles, and the little boy would smack his hand down on the bed in frustration. He re-grabbed the controller and started again. And again, Sonic got whacked, and lost his rings. This pattern continued a few more times and, finally, the frustrated little boy thrust the controller into the blanket and raised his hands and reeled off a rapid series of animated, ASL gesticulations. In the course of his angry, rapid-fire sign language, I recognized one sign alone amidst the many others: Middle and ring finger down with pinky and pointer up and thumb extended out to the side. The love sign. Or sustained by itself to someone else, "I love you." I wasn't sure what the whole context was, but I mentioned to the mom that in all that expression, the only thing I recognized was the love sign. How did that fit in? She laughed and said that he had essentially said that "This game doesn't love me and I can't win."

Certainly, a lamentation felt by many modern kids!

Sadly, that was the last time I saw the little boy. And it was about six months later that I heard that he had passed away. I assumed that another bout of pneumonia or something had been responsible. A heart-rending loss for all who had known him, but still a wonderful human accomplishment for the family who had sustained him, and who had enabled his brief stay in this universe to be the best it could be. As we ponder our own mortality, especially after many decades, it is hard to imagine one who only gets a little over five years. In this special case, he was one old enough to perceive everything about himself, knowing that he was afflicted, knowing that he needed tubes and machines while others did not, but yet, still actively partaking in the love and joy and company of those closest to him. His was a life so short, yet filled with memories of snuggling by a camp fire, seeing stars at night, catching a fish on a line, throwing rocks and wading barefoot in the water. However brief, forever precious.

The Glory to Shine a Second Time. Lung Transplantation, Organ Donation and The Gift of Life

As a homecare respiratory therapist and a Community College Instructor, I have had many opportunities not only to work with lung transplant patients, both before and after their surgeries, but also to have them come to the classroom and to share their personal experience with respiratory therapy students. I have also put on public demonstrations with lung transplant patients at medical conventions and health fairs and the like. Given the trials and tribulations that the typical transplant patient has endured, in the process of being given a second chance at life, they often want to share their experience and to express their thankfulness. Inextricably bound to that experience is the brutal reality that, for every successful transplant patient, one family's agonizing, mortal tragedy had become their personal ecstatic reprieve. Organ donation and transplantation is a multifaceted, disconcerting topic that has the potential to raise the human spirit and to bring tears to the eyes, but, at the same time, the life-and-death dynamic can be hard for many to contemplate and to assimilate. In lieu of that, arranging the opportunity to get the entire picture of the heartbreaking and yet inspirational process before a public, non-medical audience can be difficult.

At one well-attended public health-and-wellness fair at the college, I had reserved a large media room just off the main booth area for the presentation. I had a big sign-up, and lots of brochures and handouts on organ donation, and I also stood at the doorway, trying to encourage the many passers-by to join us. But as the clock ticked down, we had very few takers. I then went on the overhead intercom, to announce that the Lung Transplant presentation with our special guest speaker was starting in ten minutes and we hoped to invite as many as we could. I intimated that it would be an uplifting and motivational experience. The large meandering and milling audience however, remained unmotivated - perhaps "squeamish" would be a fairer term. I learned that organ transplantation (however potentially fascinating a topic) doesn't immediately sell well outside the classroom or medical convention environments. Maybe it is something that most people don't want to think about, as they are exploring booths laden with vitamin therapies, dietary advice, homeopathic alternative medicines, and many other wellness topics. Which of course, speaks to my choice of venue as well. At the last moment, I rounded up several current and former students, as well as coworkers from the respiratory and nursing departments, to provide a decent semblance of an audience for our special speaker.

For me, it was one of those frustrating mental situations where the old Biblical adage "if they only knew" gnawed at the mind. If they would *just get in here*! *Just see it once*! They would probably be far more inspired than they ever guessed! Ultimately, each transplant patient's story is entirely unique, as are the circumstances that favored them over someone else on the transplant list. The biggest heartache of all is realizing that a solid half of the people waiting for transplant surgery will not receive their organs in time. The following story montages (with pertinent whimsical titles) will serve briefly to chronicle the history and highlights of the three lung transplant patients with whom I had made public demonstrations, Diane, Sheila and Ed. Each story is an aggregate of personal puzzle pieces, chronologically mish-mashed somewhat, that collectively contribute to the larger picture of the lung transplant experience. For me, I experienced the transitional spectacle of first working with them privately at home, as downtrodden, decrepit, end-stage oxygen patients, and then sharing a stage with them publicly, as joyful, vibrant and active advocates after the fact. To experience the before and after up close, was beyond amazing, and, in the case of Sheila, especially, the transition was stupefying! But first, some quick background on Lung Transplantation, and some specifics on the presentations themselves.

Loosely, the history of Human Lung Transplant surgery goes back several decades, technically to the early 1960's, when a voluntary, experimental, lung transplant was performed on a life-sentence prisoner; he died eighteen days later. But the routinely successful practice of it (if you will) is quite a recent development, stemming from the mid 1980's; and it has improved remarkably further still since. Originally, only a few medical centers around the U.S. and the world provided the service, but now there are numerous centers around the country and the world doing lung transplants. When I was a student in 1976, I read an article about the difficulties in experimental lung transplants performed on dogs; alongside many other complications, the dogs typically rejected their lungs within a month. The doubtful consensus was that it was the better part of impossible that human lung transplants would ever be routinely performed in the same manner as heart and kidney transplants. The complexity and difficulties were just too numerous to overcome. Even with preparation, the mushy, spongy lungs degraded rapidly outside of the body; there were too many critical vessels and tubes to stitch together; ultimately there were too many things to go wrong. Well, time and tremendous devotion to the science and art of transplant surgery have put those negative lamentations to rest. And one of the major contributors to this thoracic art is the University of Washington in Seattle.

Given the university's proximity to where I work and live, the Transplant PowerPoint Presentations that I put together celebrate the University of Washington's Lung Transplant Program. Each presentation is templated around the UW Video: *New Lungs: The Gift of Life*, which highlights Dr. Mulligan, Dr Raghu, et al., and the entire UW transplant team of nurses, social workers, physical therapists, respiratory therapists, etc. All of these wonderful folks appearing on screen were directly involved with the care of each of the lung transplant speakers. The very real *family* element that the UW transplant team maintains with their patients, both before and after the surgery, was brought to life on stage, as the transplant patients themselves would often (during the Q&A) refer back to the specific people in the video who had assisted them with various aspects at different stages of the truly overwhelming lung transplant process.

The video was preceded by a preliminary introduction with the stated goals being *to Inform, to Encourage* and, *to Inspire*—to inform the people about the dreaded pulmonary disease at hand, to encourage them to consider organ donation themselves, and to inspire them with the story of our special speaker. Leading up to the video, the specific lung disease and its signs, symptoms and occurrence were outlined. After the video, the speaker would chronicle his or her life from childhood, all the way up to the night of *the call*! Then they talked about the surgical process itself (including some dry runs) and then the recovery process, and then they discussed the very personal details on how their lives changed (or didn't have to change) after their transplant surgery. And then we finished up with an open, even sometimes rousing question and answer session.

All aspects of these presentations were well received by the audiences at hand, except for the one following facetious exception that is contained in our first story about Diane.

Diane's story. Go Dawgs! And the flight of the hummingbird.

Alpha-1 Antitrypsin Deficiency

For die-hard Washington Husky Fans, this upcoming Alpha-1 Antitrypsin Deficiency moment is just for you. In the Spring of 2011, I worked for a homecare company called Care Medical (now gone with the DME wind), which was headquartered in Portland, Oregon. Each June, we had an annual summit at the Portland Double Tree Inn, and we partook in technical classes sponsored by CPAP and ventilator manufacturing reps, and there were academic speakers who had presentations for CEU credits and so forth. Well, coincidentally, at the time, Diane (the Alpha-1 transplant patient for whom the original presentation had been fashioned), had relocated from the Tacoma area to the Portland area. So I arranged to put on her transplant presentation for the company summit. She had been a Care Medical oxygen patient for several years and she just *barely did make the call* for her transplant surgery a couple years earlier. And I mean just barely! She had deteriorated, to the point of requiring two, ten-liter oxygen concentrators wired together to keep her oxygen levels just edging in the survivable range. Without exaggeration, she was weeks if not days from dying when the call to UW came. Diane was well known to our clinicians and customer service staff, but now that she didn't require our oxygen services any more, and that she had recently moved away, it was also an opportunity for us to get reacquainted and to share in her success.

As it turned out, on the very morning of the scheduled presentation, Diane got a call from the UW team. They had performed some tests earlier in the week, and just for precautionary purposes, they wanted her to come up to the university for a bronchoscopy procedure. So now, suddenly northbound to Seattle, Diane wasn't able to attend the Portland presentation, but we still held one in her honor. I placed an empty chair before the audience and explained the last-minute development, but we would proceed as if she were here. And certainly, she was in spirit. Also, we would still have a question and answer session at the end, since I knew her story well at this point. So, I started the presentation.

It was during the overview of the distribution and occurrence of the Alpha-1 disease, that I stumbled onto the realization that I was in foreign environs. My well-worn spiel was that Alpha-1 was common enough to devastate many families every year, yet rare enough that it continues to mostly remain off the public's radar screen. It seems that no one has ever heard of it. The occurrence of the severe form is around one in three thousand people.

And as I further related, to add some context... "if there are sixty thousand people in Husky Stadium, about twenty people in the crowd have the devastating disease and don't know it yet."

As soon as I said Husky Stadium, a low-level "boooooh" emanated from a few in the audience. Seemed odd and out of place all of a sudden.

Then it hit me. That's right. I didn't realize it. I was south of the border! Here I was, talking *"Dawgie"* in the quacky, derelict precincts of Duckville. (I hate it when that happens.) I decided to roll with the mildly impertinent flow for a moment. I said, "OK. I get it. When in Rome... let's change to your venue...if you had sixty thousand people in Autzen Stadium..." Then I paused and said, "but wait a minute... you can't even fit sixty thousand people into Autzen Stadium." Some guffaws came out, and I said, "look, the ratio is one in three thousand. You can do your own math for Autzen Stadium. And let's face it. Unlike Wazzu fans, I know you can do the math."

Purple and Gold to the end, Diane, of course (God rest her soul), was a huge UW Husky fan herself and got a big kick out of the exchange when I told her about it.

To briefly elucidate the nature of this disease, Alpha-1 Antitrypsin Deficiency is caused by a genetic lack of a protective protein (enzyme blocker) that protects body cells from the body's own defense department. The way the body goes about killing germs is a risky, kind of backwards process. When white blood cells attack germs, they release powerful digestive enzymes (called trypsin, a.k.a. neutrophil elastase) that rip and tear into a germ's protein structures. The problem is, trypsin enzymes have no capacity to distinguish friend or foe. Once released at the site of the infection, they will rip into body cells as readily as a germ cell. Well, you may wonder, incredulous, who came up with this stupid defense plan? Actually, given the tight quarters and the billions of cells in any body tissue, the process was inevitable. There is no safe place for body cells to take cover during a war with intruders. The back-door remedy is provided by the liver. The liver produces a protective protein (*anti*-trypsin) that body cells use to ward off the enzymes during a battle. As long as the body cells in the battle zone have their supply of antitrypsin, the defense department can have at it, and when the smoke and dust clears, the enemies are vanquished and the happy villagers are safe. But if the body has little to no antitrypsin production, the body tissues are now vulnerable to repeated friendly-fire damage and destruction. The reason Alpha-1 so heavily manifests in the lungs is because the lungs are the most heavily defended organ in the body. Most body organs hum along day-to-day with little defense department activity. But the lungs, being the only internal organ that is open to the outside world, take in debris, dust and germs every day, and even absent a major infection, there is mop-up duty by white blood cells going on all the time. Here, there and everywhere, this friendly-fire damage accumulates, and, since the spongy mass of the lung itself has no sensory neurons, there is no pain associated with the ongoing tissue destruction. Typically, and cruelly, by the time the thirty-five to forty-five-year-old victim suddenly develops enough shortness of breath symptoms to require a trip to the doctor, the damage done is already severe, and they will require a lung transplant in order to survive.

(People often ask if Alpha-1 is an autoimmune disease. The answer is that Alpha-1 is as close as you can get *without its being* an autoimmune disease. In an autoimmune disease, like Sheila's Polymyositis, the defense department is deliberately attacking and inflaming the body's own tissue cells. Somehow the tissue cells got marked as an enemy, and they are treated as intruders. In Alpha-1, the defense department is going about its normal, germ-killing business appropriately, and the lack of the protective protein accounts for the *friendly fire* damage.)

As a final clinical perspective, without going too deep into the weeds on it, there are many genetic variants of the disease, called phenotypes. Some are worse than others. (The perfectly normal phenotype is MM.) Arranged in order of increasing severity (i.e. deficiency of the protein), the common altered phenotypes are—MS, MZ, SS, SZ and ZZ. Diane had the dreaded ZZ phenotype, which is the critical, most deficient form of the genetic disease. But as with so many aspects of medicine and disease, the misery is not spread evenly or fairly. Growing up, Diane was the little go-getter in the family, always into athletics; she never smoked, she never drank, but she got hit hard by the disease. Ironically, she had an older sister who also was born with the ZZ phenotype—and she did drink and she did smoke, and she did eventually manifest COPD symptoms later in life, commensurate with those typical for a smoker, but not in the full, brutal Alpha-1 fashion that had devastated Diane. I have just enough incidental knowledge on the matter to mention it in passing, but there is a current theory that certain normal flora in the body may act to protect the lungs in some afflicted people. Research continues on that. As a final pathological aspect, Alpha-1 causes the lungs to erode, to thin out, to enlarge and bubble up in pure emphysema fashion. To distinguish it from other forms of emphysema, it is commonly nicknamed *genetic emphysema.*

From an interpersonal standpoint, random events often create an affinity between people, and for Diane and myself it involved hummingbirds. One winter, less than a year before her transplant surgery, with heavy snow on the ground, I went to Diane's house to experiment with a different nasal oxygen device. She had had the twin, ten-liter concentrators set up recently, and the high oxygen flowrate through the cannula was abrading her nares and nostrils. An oxygen mask would be the most appropriate device for such a high flowrate, but it made her claustrophobic. I tried fitting her with a nasal cup device to lessen the irritation to the skin. As I sat at her dining room table, adjusting the device to her face, there was movement beyond the glass doors to my right, and I turned my head. Outside above the snow-covered patio two hummingbirds swirled around each other in an aerial dogfight near a hanging feeder. Hummingbirds? In the snow? Since when? Weren't these guys supposed to be sipping Margaritas in Acapulco by now?

Diane noted that they were Anna's, a species that lived year-round in Washington state. I really couldn't remember the last time I had seen a hummingbird. I do remember the first time—it happened when I was in the first grade, walking home from school. It buzzed past my head and hovered by some tall flowers nearby. I thought it was a giant bumble bee at first, but then I realized, hey, that's a hummingbird. Cool. But now I hadn't seen a humming bird in years. Especially in winter. Diane assured me that, if you put out a feeder, they will show up out of nowhere. *Build it, and they will come!* She even gave me her own homemade recipe for the liquid food. So I took her up on it, and said that my young daughter and I would make a project out of it. Well, Diane was right. We put one feeder in the backyard, and one in front. Within five to six days, in the dead of winter, we acquired a routine visitation of hummingbirds. The feeders, of course, are still in place, some eight years later.

Post-surgery, when Diane and I made our inaugural Transplant Presentation, in front of the respiratory class, it all went splendidly, and the students made me proud, as they asked many thoughtful and worthwhile questions. In the end, after much applause, I then announced that I had a special gift for Diane. My daughter, a decently accomplished artist, had painted a rustic, rectangular wood-framed, wood-surfaced picture. The frame and background were solid white, with bright, long-hanging Fuchsia flowers, and a pair of Anna's hummingbirds hovering in place. I told the class the story of the hummingbirds at her home, and my own.

In epilogue, here, the most piercing Diane moment, for me, thankfully, didn't last long. My favorite service tech-oxygen driver of all time is a guy named John. He is an Iowa native. No finer gentleman will you meet: a rock climber, a fisherman, a mountain hiker. He and I shared many conversations over the years. He and Diane were good friends, also, and, actually, his service rounds took him to Diane's house more often than did mine. But he would routinely update me on her condition whenever he had had recent contact with her. One day, I happened to be up in the warehouse by the truck bay, when John wheeled two ten-liter concentrators off his truck lift and pushed them in, side-by-side. Ten-liter oxygen concentrators are rarely set up by themselves, much less to have two of them at once. As he got closer, sure enough, they looked just like the ones at the house. As John came up, I asked anxiously, already knowing the answer:

"Whose are those?"

John affirmed, "They're Diane's."

I just stared blankly at them for a moment, and John asked, "Didn't you hear?"

I responded flatly, forlorn. "No, I didn't hear." Looking up, I couldn't understand why John was smirking.

Knowing what I was thinking, he grinned even more and said, happily, "She got her lung transplant."

Sheila's story.
"As long as you have breath, there is hope."
And the Clash of the Sibling Beauties

Polymyositis with Pulmonary Invasion.

Sheila's story is especially close to home, because she is the older sister of a wonderful customer service lady named Jessica, with whom I had worked for several years. Sheila had languished on the lung transplant list for quite a while, but I never got to know her until very late in the going. Even though her sister worked for our homecare company, Sheila didn't come on to our oxygen services, because we were not contracted with her insurance company plan. As time went by, her condition quickly worsened, but she was a determined fighter, and tried to maintain her personal independence for as long as possible. Then one of her doctors suggested that she get a portable oxygen concentrator, to see if it would aid her better in getting around. So he wrote a prescription for one. It turned out that her existing homecare company did not carry POCs, so, in that case, her insurance was open to getting one from an alternate, out of network source. Since we were one of the few DME (durable medical equipment) companies that specialized in POCs, we were happy that we could at least do something for Jessica's sister.

My first meeting with Sheila was at her apartment, for the POC set up. Sheila suffered from an autoimmune disease called Polymyositis (*many muscle inflammations*). And unlike the sinister, silent, and painless Alpha-1 or IPF, Polymyositis can have episodes of extreme body pain, sometimes felt on the skin as if the body is on fire, and, other times, deep focal pain, like horrible muscle cramps, only there is no actual cramp, and, if you dare to try to rub the area, the pain intensifies. At times Sheila found herself lying on the floor, screaming in pain, yet pleading that no one touch her! It is a wretchedly cruel, and torturing disease. Polymyositis is rather rare, and traditionally difficult to diagnose. Like many sufferers, Sheila had spent a long time going to different doctors, and taking different medications until it was finally properly diagnosed. More rarely still does it attack the lungs and facilitate fibrotic scarring, and more rarely still does it (apparently) contribute to pulmonary hypertension. But Sheila had all of this! It was a lot of medical misery to pack into one woman's body. Much remains unknown about Polymyositis (and its whole family of related autoimmune disorders), but Sheila's devastating trifecta combination was thought to occur on the order of one in *numerous millions* of people.

When I first saw Sheila at her apartment, it was a heartbreaking sight. She was tremendously shriveled and emaciated. This vicious disease had wreaked its havoc upon her. Her face was bony, and her eyes were sunken like those of a severely starving person. At the same time, her taut facial skin had an almost raisin-like texture to it, as if she had been bodily placed into a dehydrator. And owing to her withdrawn facial features, her large white teeth protruded from her retracted lips. I felt so sorry for her. The cruelty and indignity of this consuming disease was on full display.

(Over a year later, after her surgery, during a reunion between a large group of transplant patients and their beloved surgeon, Dr. Michael Mulligan, he had told Sheila that, of all the transplant patients he had worked with, she was the most concerning of all. He had his serious doubts. By the time of her surgery, she was so shriveled and emaciated, he feared that she might not have enough strength left—enough physical and mental oompah!—to pull herself through the tough, post-operative process. But oh, did she ever!)

As it turned out, that day at the apartment, the battery operated POC didn't have enough oompah either. It didn't elevate her oxygen saturation well enough at all. Her degraded condition and her high oxygen needs had outstripped the current technological capability of our portable devices. She had to stay with her cumbersome, heavy oxygen cylinders, and soon she was pretty much housebound. She languished many more months like this, until her call to transplant came.

I wasn't immediately informed about her transplant when it happened, but within weeks she had made a roaring recovery. And, one day, I walked out of my office and out into the company show room area. I saw that Jessica was at the counter with a customer, so I walked over to see if she needed me to get her anything. As I came up and stood there, Jessica was brandishing her bright smile, and sweetly yakking it up with the customer. The customer had an equally radiant smile and beaming face.

As I stood there, the two finished their chipper exchange, then the lady at the counter looked directly at me and said eagerly, "Hi!"

I looked back and responded, a little reserved, "Hi".

Then she started laughing, and leaned over toward me. She squealed, "You don't know who I am, do you?"

I stammered, "uhm... well...". Then Jessica started squealing.

The lady said, "I'm Sheila!"

And even after she said Sheila, I still paused for a second. She added, "I got my double lung transplant."

Stupefied, all I could say was "Wow!" I felt embarrassed, and I felt displaced for not recognizing her, and the ladies could tell that I was stymied by her dramatic change in appearance, and it made them squeal even more. Nothing in my memory bank could have connected the pathetic, shriveled face in the apartment several months back, with the ravishing, lively woman standing before me now. I remembered a tragically-stricken face from some third world disaster, and now I was looking at a glowing, Kerry Washington-Jennifer Hudson, African-American beauty queen. And she had the shnazz and the jazz in her persona to go with her looks, too. I was dumbfounded. (We will address Sheila's actual age upcoming. But she could easily pass for thirty-something.)

Then Jessica chided, "Yeah, she looks good after her surgery. But I was always the prettiest in the family."

Sheila dished it right back, "Give it up, little girl. You lived in my shadow your whole life!"

Big sis' and little sis' dished it back and forth, and, for me, it was pure enchantment. What a phenomenal difference a new set of lungs can make! The total rejuvenation of this woman was glorious to behold.

After mixing it up with Jessica, I told Sheila that I wanted to run something by her, so we went into my office. I told her about the lung transplant presentations that I had been doing with Diane, and now that Diane had relocated, I was on hiatus for the moment. I asked if she had any desire to do some public presentations herself. And she was more than game for that. She had already gone back to UW once to talk to her former compatriots, who were still on the waiting list. She wanted to offer them some hope and encouragement. She remembered being on the waiting list herself, and having successful transplant survivors come back and do the same. And now she wanted to get out in public, and encourage people to become organ donors. So, it was all a go. We would fashion a new presentation around polymyositis, and Sheila would put her personal story in order on paper, and then we would make a slide show out of it.

Shortly thereafter, Sheila called upon one of the major members of the UW transplant team - a renowned social worker named Angela - to assist her with getting the right words and the right ways to express herself, and to promote the UW program as well. As insanely busy as Angela's daily job is, she was kind enough to put together a list of encouraging tips and techniques, and she included some

UW program highlights, including the fact that the very first UW lung transplant patient from the early nineties was still alive!

Several weeks later, our first presentation was in the classroom, before the respiratory therapy students at the college. She was a big hit. Everyone fell in love with her, and the girls in the class all came running up to hug her at the end. And speaking of affection and good looks and what not, somehow you can't do a UW Lung Transplant Video presentation without addressing the dashing and debonair countenance of Dr. Michael Mulligan. I never initiated the topic, but it came up in both Diane's and Sheila's presentations in the classroom. In the past, Diane had assured the girls in class that (believe it or not), "he's even more handsome in person than he is on screen!" Today, Sheila summed it up succinctly, "He's a *hottie*, ladies!" All in good fun.

During Sheila's recounting of her personal experiences that day in class, she talked about the one dry run she had. Several patients have had this happen, where you get "the call" and make a safe but mad rush to the university hospital; you get all prepped up and ready to go, and you end up spending several anxious hours in waiting, only to have it scrubbed, due to some last-minute technicality. It was a huge emotional roller coaster ride to endure in a single day. In her case, the call came in the morning, before breakfast, so her girlfriend came right over and helped her to lug her oxygen cylinders into the car and off they went, North on I-5. At the hospital, she got swooped up into a flurry of activity, and then the whole day dragged on until well after sun down, and then it was finally declared a "no-go." A dry run. Time to pack it all up and go home.

Well, Sheila was not only dog-tired after all that, but she had not eaten anything since the night before! They had taken off before breakfast and it was now after dinnertime. She was starving! She said she was hungrier than she had ever been in her life. On the way back in the car Sheila was desperately searching ahead for a fast-food place. Any place. Her favorite was Jack-in the-Box and lo and behold, they saw Jack just ahead! Salvation! Jack, my man! Hurry, hurry! They pulled up, hopped right out, and Sheila dragged her oxygen tank inside and up to the counter and ordered just a Jumbo Jack. When the counterman handed it to her she ripped the wrapper open and attacked the burger mercilessly, as the counterman looked on, aghast. Bite after bite, not finishing one before she ripped off another. Sheila looked up at him and said, between chews, "I know this looks bad. . .but I haven't eaten since yesterday... got tied up all today with something important... but it didn't happen... too much to explain."

As a signature sendoff, at the end of this first presentation before the class, Sheila expressed her personal, passionate refrain, for all those waiting on the transplant list, "As long as you have breath, there is hope."

About a year later, at an inaugural College Respiratory Convention, Sheila and I went before the largest audience to date. We were positioned as the grand finale of sorts. Standing at the lectern, I introduced Sheila, seated in a chair to my left. She looked sweet and svelte, in her black form-fitting pants and black sweater top. Now, it may seem distracting and gratuitous for me to keep addressing her physical appearance, but there was a method to my seemingly-ogling madness. It gave me an opportunity to drive an important aspect home to the audience. A lot of people think of transplant surgery as a stop-gap, patch-the-fuselage-with-beer-cans-and-keep-the-old-plane-flying kind of thing. Transplants may keep you alive, but are you really *living* afterward? Aren't you mostly half of your former self? Many have the idea that you end up lumbering around, all stitched up like Frankenstein, and taking a thousand medications a day. And really, what kind of life is that? Well, if there were any Frankenstein sentiments in the audience that night, Sheila incinerated them.

So, toward the end of my introduction, I drew attention to Sheila's countenance. Initially, I told the audience that we were going to explore Polymyositis and what a truly mentally and physically devastating disease it was.

I told them about the first time I saw her in the apartment, and how shriveled up she was, and how sorry I had felt for her.

I told them that she had so greatly deteriorated, by the time of her call to transplant, that her surgeon worried that she would not survive the transplant surgery itself.

But obviously, she did.

And then I told them the story of Sheila and her little sister Jessica at the work counter, and how stymied I was that I didn't recognize her. Then I focused the audience's attention directly to Sheila.

I invited them to take a good look at her. "After all the physical misery that she had endured for years, take note of how healthy and radiant and vibrant she is."

Then I asked them, "does she look to you like a forty-two-year-old woman who was deathly sick for years, and has had a double lung transplant?"

The audience immediately responded, with expressions of kudos, nodding and gesticulating, agreeing wholeheartedly. She looked great.

I then encouraged them, "Please give this brave woman a hand for all that she has been through." The audience responded enthusiastically, clapping and cheering. As the applause dwindled and subsided, I looked over to Sheila and inquired sheepishly, "Did I lie?"

Sheila grinned her big, beautiful smile and looked at the audience and said, "Yes, he lied. I am actually sixty-two years old."

The audience jolted; gasps and sighs erupted. Nooo waaay! You got to be kidding! It really was shocking. Now they were stupefied!

Then I said to the audience, "Now you know how I felt at the counter that day!"

Then I added, "Don't let anyone tell you that life after transplant has to be a suboptimal life. You can rise to full glory again."

That night Sheila spoke from the heart, and the audience loved it. She talked about all the changes in priorities which she had. Things she used to worry about are now the furthest things from her mind. She makes it a point to enjoy each and every day. She said that she makes regular visits to the UW, to encourage other people on the list. She tells them that, *as long as you have breath, there is hope.* She said living on that list is like living in one fading world, hoping to get transported to another world. Another world that exists right around you: the one your family and loved ones live in. By the end of her stirring talk, I think many people in the crowd were willing to remove their own organs, right then and there, and donate them tonight!

We will conclude Sheila's story by returning to the night of her *second call.* She vividly recalled the dramatic details of this event and enjoyed sharing them with everyone that night. But we will revisit this event together as a supportive, real-time fly on the wall.

Outside the operating room, lying on the gurney in the surgical staging area, Sheila stared at the ceiling wondering what was going to happen...wondering how long she could keep doing this. She knew she couldn't keep this pace up much longer. She was tired, and much weaker now than ever before. This was her second chance for surgery. Maybe it would be another dry run. Maybe she would be back at Jack-in-the-Box. But that would be OK. Many of her friends on the transplant list never got a chance at all. And in just a few months, Sheila would exceed the age limit, and be bumped from the list herself. But that, too, was OK. Maybe God had other plans for her. And she was willing to accept that. She would wait and see. *As long as you have breath, there is hope.* And she still had breath. Down the hallway behind her was a communications room. The door had been left ajar, and she could now hear transmitted radio voices, talking back and forth. She starkly realized that it was the procurement team, out on location somewhere, assessing the donated lungs. She listened carefully. They were getting a final report back to the surgical department. Then she heard them announce, "Match. We got a match. It's a go... it's a go."

Tears pouring down her wrinkled, shriveled face, she repeated to herself, "It's a go! It's a go! Oh, thank you God! It's a go!"

About the only other inside sentiment to add to such a powerful moment would be, *Jessica pretty little sister—look out! For however long we can enjoy it, pretty big sister is coming baaack!*

He's number one! The Uproariously Hypoxic Life and Times of "Ex-Vivo" Ed

Idiopathic Pulmonary Fibrosis

The story of Ed is a lesson in human physical perseverance and unrelenting mental self-control. He was afflicted with Idiopathic Pulmonary Fibrosis (IPF). Paralleling Alpha-1 sufferers on a couple of accounts, people afflicted with this ferocious and silent lung disease typically live three years or less after diagnosis, unless they get a lung transplant. The difference is that IPF tends to occur a little later in life than Alpha-1 (in one's fifties, rather than the thirties and forties), and it occurs more often in males than females. The pathophysiology of this *idiopathic* ("no-known reason") fibrosis is both totally mysterious, and yet easy to relate to when compared to straightforward pulmonary fibrosis. The easiest pulmonary fibrosis for the lay person to relate to is asbestosis. Of all the materials (rock dust, mortar dust, coal dust, wood micro-particles) that can invade the lung and create a fibrosis (scarring and thickening), the most notorious is asbestos.

First of all, the lungs have a highly efficient clearance and defense system, that routinely moves particles up and out. Furthermore, over and above the standard white blood cells (neutrophils) that do most of the germ killing, there exists in the lungs a gnarly white blood cell called the Alveolar Macrophage (the "big-eater", a.k.a. Macky!) who happens to be one of the "baddest-dude" white blood cell types in the body. Neutrophils actually die in the act of killing germs, but not Macky! He gobbles germs one after another, and keeps going. A denizen of the pulmonary deep, he prowls the alveolar surfaces looking for trouble, and can easily slip into nooks and crannies between cells (i.e. third space) looking for any extra-cellular interlopers. And, if Macky happens upon a dust particle, or a pollen particle, he can eat them, too! But not even Macky can eat asbestos.

Under a microscope, fine asbestos particles look like jagged blades, with spikey edges and when they get inhaled deep into the lung, the blades get lodged into the micro sidewalls, and they stay put. If the lungs can't get rid of the foreign object by moving it upward (or having Macky eat it), the last resort is to build scar tissue over it. Over time, the asbestos-laden alveolar membranes thicken up, and it becomes increasingly difficult for oxygen to diffuse across the scar tissue and into the blood. Eventually the cartilage mass not only impedes the oxygen absorption into the blood, but it squishes and crowds out the blood flow in the vessels themselves, making everything a whole lot worse. The lungs progressively cinch up, turning leathery, and are very hard to stretch on inhalation. This increases the work of breathing over and above the two other factors of oxygen depletion. Pulmonary fibrosis, especially in its late stages, is an excruciating thing to endure. It relentlessly suffocates you into the grave. A final point: asbestosis is easy to diagnose. It's so obvious that anyone could recognize it. A lung tissue sample under a microscope clearly shows the thickened cartilage mass, laced with all the well-preserved asbestos blades, in plain sight. (But it gets worse. Unlike other inert particles, asbestos is highly chemically reactive and cancer-causing. But that is another miserable story.)

We can sum up all the devastating personal, clinical, and pathological factors by comparing the unexpected, devastating news given to each, an Alpha-1 patient and an IPF patient:

Bad news for the unwitting Alpha-1 patient: even though you couldn't feel it happening, your lungs are destroyed. Even though you've never smoked, you have the degraded, emphysema-ridden lungs of a sixty-pack-a-year smoker. All other body systems are normal and healthy, but you're going to die within three years or so if you don't get a lung transplant. The cause is an unfortunate genetic deficiency of a critical protein.

Bad news for the unwitting IPF patient: even though you couldn't feel it happening, your lungs are destroyed. You have the thickened, scarred-up lungs of an unprotected, long-term asbestos worker. Only there is no asbestos. Or any other particle material. The scar tissue is perfectly clean. We don't know why this happens. But you will die within three years or so, if you don't get a lung transplant.

You can imagine how devastating it must be for an otherwise happy healthy person to walk into the doctor's office, thinking that they may have some kind of asthma, or mild bronchitis that is making them short of breath on exertion, and then to get slammed with either one of the above scenarios.

Ed is one of these people. He was told he had IPF. He was told that he had three years to live. Somehow, against heavy odds, living in slow motion, Ed persisted for well over twice that long. And over that brutal time period, he developed an attitude and practice of avoiding all negativity. He stubbornly believed in the power of positive thinking. No matter how bad it gets, stay upbeat. He attended support groups for a while, but he found that they tended to gravitate to negative feelings, and sometimes outright anger, at the mysterious and deathly ailment that they shared. As unfair as life is, dousing yourself in negativity only makes it worse, and Ed was striving to avoid that. Stay upbeat, stay upbeat, don't let other people or your disease get you down. But sometimes, maybe inadvertently, people can get you down. And one time, given how long he had continued to live against the heavy odds, one of the many medical personnel involved in his care had made an off-handed, perhaps clumsy, inadvertent comment about it. Instead of expressing something on the order of, "it is amazing and inspiring how long you have endured this disease against the statistics, Ed," it was a more direct, and dismissive, "I can't believe you are still alive, Ed."

How exactly did he intend for Ed to take that expressive sentiment? Was he impressed with Ed's personal staying power, or was Ed just a detached example of something that conflicted with his pre-existing knowledge of the normal progress of the disease?

With just a tad more bluntness, in a callous and inverted celebration of his own knowledge on the matter, he could have gotten to the crux, "How come you're not dead, Ed?" To which Ed might have responded, "well, breath by breath, day by day. I am determined to keep putting it off."

Clinicians at any level need always to be careful of their word choices. Especially when working around terminal patients. From a human perspective, it can be awkward. What do you really say to a terminal patient? Do you try to cheer them up? Ultimately, the Hippocratic perspective works best here—whatever you say, *do no harm*. Be helpful, be polite, and perhaps resist the urge to say too much, even though real empathy may coax you in that regard. And if you do comment directly about someone's terminal illness, take some great advice from Ed's own personal Mantra—stay upbeat!

As of this moment of writing, Ed's story continues to be *singularly* unique. By definition, unique isn't supposed to carry a modifier, but the dynamic circumstances of Ed's story require it.

Going back in time, in the Spring of 2009, it was after eight p.m., and I was still languishing at the Car Pros Kia Dealer, waiting for my wife to finish squeezing one last drop of blood out of the sales manager, before finalizing the purchase of a Kia Rhondo, when my business cell rang. It was Ed. Thankfully, Ed pulled me away from the grueling business at hand. I told my wife, "I really need to take this." The sales manager had that "please don't go" look on his face, terrified of my leaving him alone with *the negotiator*.

But Ed was more important. He took priority, and I took off out of there.

Ed was calling from a restaurant in Poulsbo, WA, about fifty miles away. Planning a few nights away from town, a couple of days earlier Ed had come into our office to get a portable oxygen concentrator (POC) for the local trip. For extended trips away from home, a POC is much more convenient than a cumbersome load of oxygen cylinders. Like the large, stationary oxygen concentrators in the home, they pull in in regular air (twenty-one per cent oxygen) and run it through a sieve material that separates it from the Nitrogen (seventy-eight per cent of the air) and diverts the concentrated oxygen to a pressure tank and pumps it to the patient. The concentrated oxygen delivered is about ninety-two per cent to a maximum of ninety-six per cent purity. (Cylinder oxygen is pure one hundred per cent.) As long as you have power, you have oxygen. But if the pump inside the concentrator fails—a very rare event— all oxygen production stops cold. And, unfortunately, Ed had just become a current recipient of that technical knowledge.

Ed relayed his predicament calmly to me. The portable concentrator was dead. He did have his finger-pulse oximeter with him, and, as long as he stayed very still, his hemoglobin saturation readings were running at about eighty-six per cent, give or take a couple. With advanced IPF, if you get active at all without oxygen, your hemoglobin, oxygen saturation can plummet to life-threatening levels. And the desperate work of breathing, to try to reverse it, can become a diminishing return. The stiffened, fibrotic lungs can be so hard to stretch that the breathing muscles themselves are burning up more oxygen than can be resupplied to them—much less to the rest of the body! A horrible, suffocating downward spiral ensues. If any oxygen patient gets in dire straits anywhere at any time the rapid solution is to call 9-1-1. Ed wasn't at that 9-1-1 point yet, and was going to avoid it as best he could. I got off the phone briefly and called the on-call oxygen driver, and he made a bee-line to Poulsbo forthwith. I called Ed back, to let him know that reinforcements were on the way. It would be about an hour or a little more. So, breath by breath, minute by minute, keeping his eye on the oximeter, Ed stayed relaxed, and calmly waited for the truck to arrive...

    What makes Ed's case so interesting is that he is the first patient in UW transplant history to have his lungs procured (harvested from the donor and transported) in a whole new way. And this process also led to him having his own "Sheila moment" in the very same surgical staging area—but again, in a whole new way. And furthermore, this new process enabled us to inject a humorous dimension into the slide show, that was a lot of fun. This new method, called Ex-Vivo, has been successfully used in few places elsewhere, but the one drawback is that it is much more expensive than the standard process. (Many health insurance companies have not come fully on board in paying for it, yet.) In general, the entire hustle-bustle pace of getting lungs transplanted within four to eight hours after harvesting is inherent to the standard procedure. In simplified sequence, the lungs go from a warm body, to a cold ice cooler, and back into a warm body again.

Prominently featured in the UW video is a transplant nurse specialist named Michael, whose job it is to harvest, prepare and preserve the donated lungs in between the donor and the recipient. His vital, not-so-technical transport device is a pedestrian, blue and white Igloo ice cooler on wheels with a tow handle. (The deluxe model.) He is the highly venerated "guardian of the cooler." The Ark of the Gift of Life.

This tight window for lung transplant necessitates an enormous amount of activity to be co-ordinated in a very short period of time. To use Diane's transplant scenario as an example, she got her gift of life from a twenty-eight-year-old mother who had been tragically killed in a snowmobile accident in Montana. Both the surgeon and the procurement nurse (cooler in tow) flew to Montana in a specially outfitted Lear Jet. Diane was notified of a possible donor. Many tests were done on site, and, when a match was determined, the lungs were harvested and preserved, and as the Lear Jet wheels lifted from the runway in Montana, a flurry of activity was underway back at the University Hospital in Seattle. The surgical suite was prepared, heart lung machines and anesthesia machines were set up and staged; Diane arrived at the hospital, and was prepped and placed into the surgical staging area. This entire, urgent orchestration is hostage to the fact that lungs degrade rapidly outside of the body. Time is of the essence. You've got to get those lungs transplanted ASAP if not sooner!

Is there a better way? Perhaps a less frantic way? Maybe, a more cool, calm and collected way? Maybe...the Ed way?

As mentioned, the newer process is called Ex-Vivo, which means, "alive outside the body." In this (high-tech) living technique, the lungs go from a warm body, to a warm incubator, and back into a warm body again. And while they are in the warm, plexiglass-bubble incubator, the lungs are connected to a ventilator that gently keeps them breathing as well. At the same time, an artificial blood solution is pumped and circulated through the lungs. This facilitates normal blood flow, keeps all the micro vessels open, and likewise serves to filter and flush out all white blood cells and stray proteins that might contribute to downstream rejection. Anthropomorphically, the intended effect is to have the lungs "think-feel" that nothing has changed; they haven't gone anywhere. The biggest contributor to downstream tissue rejection is called *ischemia reperfusion inury*. In the standard method, it relates to the initial refilling of warm blood into the cool, empty lungs, perfusing the vessels and tissue like a sponge. If the "reawakening" lung tissue becomes shocked, or inflamed by the process, it can exude its own proteins and tissue hormones that, in Dr. Mulligan's own words, "will announce to the recipient that it doesn't belong there. And that will set off an immunologic avalanche...and the long-term results of the surgery are compromised." The Ex-Vivo technique is designed to pre-empt any tissue inflammation throughout the harvesting and re-implanting process. And, best of all, the lungs can be casually preserved for up to twenty-four hours or more. (You could perform four hectic standard transplants in that time period!) Ultimately, compared to the standard technique, Ex-Vivo buys a lot of time at the outset, and greatly reduces the chances of rejection down the road.

A whole lot of factors, medical, financial, tissue-match and otherwise, had contributed to Ed's long delay in getting his lung transplant. Ultimately, the corporate entity involved in producing and promoting the new Ex-Vivo process, came to make Ed an offer he couldn't refuse. If he volunteered to be the first Ex-Vivo for UW, they would cover the costs of the surgery.

Ed was end-stage IPF and beyond. He had carried this terminal burden, and had frustrated the grim reaper for a very long time. Living in perpetual slow motion, he had boldly endured what few people had ever endured before. He hadn't had a normal Oxygen Saturation in years. He had lived on the pulmonary edge, maybe just one unfortunate incident away from the IPF spiral of no return. He eagerly agreed to the offer.

In the interim, for myself, Ed had been an oxygen patient of ours for years. Periodically I would be at the office when he came in. I always enjoyed talking with him. My buddy, John, the oxygen driver, got to know him well, also. He was just one of those straight-up, thoughtful people, of which this world of ours is in such short supply. He never pitied himself at all. He never thought of himself as a victim. As the disease progressed, he dealt with the issues as best he could. Commonly experienced by IPF victims, the range of normal daily activities begin to clue you in to the advancement of the disease over time. For rhetorical example, already resigned to living in slow motion, it used to be that you could push the shopping cart down two aisles, before having to stop and rest. Then it becomes one aisle. Then half an aisle. Then you quit shopping altogether. Soon these stifling limitations creep in through the walls of your home. Do I walk non-stop to the bathroom? Or do I rest once along the way? I remember Ed's detailing these kinds of necessary preoccupations. With IPF, you really need to plan out your activities in advance, and to provide a lot more time cushion than you ever would have had to provide in the past. And speaking of time, I distinctly remember pondering a few times, where it occurred to me, that I hadn't seen nor heard about Ed in quite a while. But one fine day, in a reversal of the Diane moment, John came up to me waving a service order, and said, "Guess where I'm going?"

I just waited in anticipation, and he proclaimed exuberantly, "I'm picking up Ed's oxygen equipment. He got his transplant!"

Yes! This was awesome news! I fished around for a post-it note. I wrote my personal cell number on it, and asked John to give it to him. "Ask Ed, at his convenience, when he's up to it, if he could give me a call. I need to talk to the boy!"

On the day when Ed got *the call* to surgery, his wife drove him up to the UW Medical Center. Ed got whisked in and prepped, and his wife was permitted to accompany him into the surgical staging area. It was the same area where Sheila (God rest her magnificent soul) had heard the radio communication some five years earlier. Ed's *Sheila moment* was entirely visual, instead of auditory. While lying there, talking with his wife, and saying a few prayers, Ed looked over to the side where some equipment tables were parked. At first, he wasn't sure what he was looking at, and then it became strangely obvious. Atop one of the tables was a plexiglass bubble. Inside were two pink lungs, slowly expanding and contracting, seemingly on their own. A nurse had stepped in bedside, and Ed asked if those were his? The nurse looked over, and was obviously startled to see the Ex-Vivo operating in full view. She said to Ed, "I am not sure if you were supposed to see that beforehand, but...yes, those are yours." Ed said he didn't feel freaked out by it at all. He actually felt a sense of comfort, the sense of a great struggle finally coming to an end. He would deal with thoughts about the donor at a later time. For posterity, Ed's wife pulled out her smart phone and took a video of the lungs in the bubble. And we later incorporated that video into Ed's slide presentation as well.

Ed's first presentation before the respiratory students was a humorous combination of technical, clinical, social, and lifestyle issues. Regarding Ex-Vivo, we had a slide of a Lear Jet flying high among the clouds. The next slide displayed the ceremonial blue and white Igloo Cooler. The following slide showed the same Lear Jet with the cooler photoshopped on top of it—zooming back to the UW Medical Center. Go, go, go! Exciting and dramatic as it was, that was the old way! Enter now, the new way. The next series of slides showed diagrams and pictures of the Ex-Vivo process and its many components. And then the initial climax was the showing of the "lungs in the bubble." The very lungs he carried inside him today.

Ed's hospital stay was chronicled in pictures as well. His wife captured the image of him in his bed, on a ventilator, moments after his return from surgery. Then she captured herself with him as he was first awake and alert. Then there were pictures of his initial rehabilitation, standing in the hall with a physical therapist, leaning on a rolling support frame, attached to a trellis of IV tubes and two sets of chest tube systems, one for each lung. It was mind-boggling.

Finally, the question and answer session went on for a long time, as Ed was full of humorous micro-instructions on how to avoid infections on every issue from flu shots, diet, travel, hand-washing, and so forth. He had to protect his new lungs, for sure, but he didn't want to be a total, germophobic freak about it, either. He would cut himself some slack here and there, splurge on few things now and then, but day-old sushi was not one of them!

We will finish Ed's incredible journey by going back into time... back to the restaurant in Poulsbo, in the Spring of 2009, where he sat with his broken concentrator, waiting for the oxygen truck to arrive. It was, no doubt, a very long hour for him. Breath by breath, minute by minute. As deteriorated as he already was, little did he know, that the conditions that would lead to his double lung transplant were still a long way off in time. And one has to wonder: if he had known in advance how long it would be, would it have crushed his spirit? Would it have sapped his stubborn strength? Would he have thrown in the towel? Sometimes it is better not to know such things in advance. Sitting there in the Spring of 2009, the circumstances that would finally coalesce and get him his new set of lungs, his new gift of life, were not destined to materialize until the summer of 2014, well over five miserable years into the future. Deteriorated as he was, it would seem frankly impossible that—breath by breath, minute by minute, day by day—he could ever so have outstripped the odds, and have dragged his IPF across such a physically and spiritually crushing gauntlet of time.

Maybe, in the final analysis, looking back on that torturous, long and winding road, all careless and maladroit comments aside, maybe it wouldn't be inappropriate after all, for a thoroughly thoughtful, and deeply compassionate person to throw their arms up and to ask, in true, sincere, wonderment, "How come you're not dead, Ed?"

Obituary

Michael William Cline was born on January 25, 1956 in Alexandria, Virginia, and passed away unexpectedly at the age of 62 from a heart attack on March 10, 2018. Mike was raised in Tacoma, Washington, and was a graduate of Bellarmine High School, Class of 1974. He would later go on to get his Bachelor's of Health Science in Professional Development and Advanced Patient Care from Grand Canyon University. He entered the healthcare field as a Respiratory Therapist, and he provided respiratory services to many different patients over the years while working for American HomePatient, Care Medical, Norco, and Performance Home Medical. He was also a lead instructor in the RT Program at Tacoma Community College, where he taught hundreds of students over the course of many years.

    Mike was a devoted husband and a loving father, and anyone who knew him personally would say that he was a selfless individual who proudly put the needs and happiness of others far before his own. He was a man of many talents, and his greatest hobbies included woodstrip boat building, fishing, storytelling, automotive repair, political analysis, deep fry cooking, bird watching, nature hiking, narrative and educational writing, and he was even the author of two published books, one on boat building and the other on respiratory care.

Mike was a true gift to all who knew him and he will be dearly missed. His memory and legacy are fondly cherished by his loving wife Tara Cline, and his beloved children Christopher and Kaela Cline. He is preceded in death by his parents, William and Sarah (Sally) Cline, and his departed brother Richard (Dick) Cline. He has three surviving brothers; Thomas, Andy and John Cline, two step brothers; Mike and Tommy Nelson, and two sisters; Anna Cline and Mary Stevens. He was loved and treasured by many more people, too numerous to mention.

A celebration of life service was held at Mountain View Funeral Home in the Aspen Chapel in Lakewood, Sunday, March 18th at 11:30 am, with a subsequent reception. There was also a public viewing from 10:00 am to 6:00 pm on Saturday, March 17th. Remembrances may be shared for family and friends at www.mountainviewtacoma.com.

AFTERWORD

Thank you very much for taking the time to read through my father's memoir. I hope that it was an enlightening and an endearing experience, one that will hopefully have a profound impact upon your own journey through the world of respiratory care, or otherwise within the proverbial Ocean of Air.

As has no doubt been evident from Michael Cline's many different stories, my father lived a very profound and eventful life. His passion for respiratory care was only matched by his love for writing and telling stories. However, both were still vastly small when compared to his tremendous love for the people that he served throughout his life. Words cannot do his genuine, selfless, good-hearted nature the justice that it deserves, but if this much love was put into bettering the lives of others entrusted in his care, one can probably only scarcely imagine the amount of love and care he put into raising both my sister Kaela and I. As I stated in my foreword, he truly was the greatest man that I have ever known.

While I unfortunately did not get the chance to know my grandfather, the "ineffable Bill Cline", very well before his passing, my childhood was full of stories about him and the many experiences he shared between my father and his many siblings, and my own life was also quite full of its own fair share of "hospital, dinner-table talk". And, just like my grandfather, my father emphatically encouraged me to get an actual skill in addition to an education, albeit perhaps a bit more lovingly! While my own passions and personal career path led more into video producing and production coordination work in the entertainment industry, my father's dedication to learning, obligation to quality, and commitment to kindness remain to be the greatest sources of inspiration in my life.

Some of my greatest childhood memories, though I didn't know it at the time, were those late-night occasions where my sister and I would have to accompany my father on a last-minute equipment setup, or an on-call CPAP emergency that needed his attention, because the two of us were too young to be left home alone. Even as a young boy I knew my father was very special, and that he knew more about "breathing air" than I would ever even hope to come close to understanding. I'll never forget the times spent driving to hospitals with him, or helping load up his car with the respiratory equipment that he needed to bring to a patient's house. As my father changed companies over the years, from American HomePatient, to Care Medical, to Norco, and to finally Performance Home Medical, one factor always remained consistent: He was irreplaceable when he left! No one ever could quite match the skillset and charm of Respiratory Therapist Michael Cline, or just "Dad" as my sister and I always called him, and his irreplaceability has only been compounded now that he has left this world for the next.

As a very grateful son, who was blessed beyond measure to have had Michael Cline as my father, I very humbly make a request to you, the reader, to in some small way help to spread the word about this book. Whether it's a positive review on Amazon, a short and sweet recommendation on your social media page describing what you learned, or even something as simple as sharing the book with a friend or colleague. My father's legacy in the world of respiratory care will continue for as long as there are people out there who are willing to learn from his experiences, and who choose to embody the traits that made him who he was. It is my fondest hope that one day that this book may indeed be read by every single respiratory therapist in the world, and perhaps even incorporated into some form of required reading in every sort of respiratory therapy educational program.

After all, there is not a person alive who would not benefit from having Michael Cline as a part of their lives. God willing, and with your help, hopefully more and more people will get the opportunity. And again, thank you very much for taking the time to read it for yourself.

Christopher M. Cline

In Memory of My Pwa-Pwa

Dear Dad,

Words truly cannot describe how much my family and I miss you. Ever since the day of your passing, there has been a hole left in my heart that I am afraid will never again be filled.

However, it is during this tragic time that I am able to find great comfort in reflecting on the special things you have taught and instilled in me, and I can continue to live on holding onto all of the beautiful and wonderful memories that were created because of you. I certainly could not be the person that I am today if it was not for all of the love, attention, and support that you provided me throughout all the days of my life.

Thank you for being the devoted husband to Mom, and the caring father to my brother and I that you always were. Thank you for being there for my family when times got tough. Thank you for teaching me to be patient and strong when life's obstacles arose, and for guiding me through these challenging times when stresses appeared too large to handle on my own. Thank you for teaching me to never lose faith or to give up on my dreams. Thank you for all of the time you dedicated to bettering my education through homeschooling my brother and I, and for doing everything in your power to set us both up for success in life. Thank you for continuously striving to put the needs of the family so far before your own and for always going the extra mile to ensure that we were all living to our full potential.

    Lastly, thank you for just being you; the most loving father that I am so incredibly blessed to have been able to call my own. I honestly could not have asked for a more perfect father, and you will forever be my rock, my protector, my friend, and my hero. The memories that I carry today I will cherish forever and ever, and although your presence may appear to be gone now, I know that you are still watching over all of us and that there will come a day when we will be back together again…

I love you with all of my heart Pwa-Pwa,

Love,
Kaela (your Gricky)